ONE STEP FURTHER

One Step Further

STEVE GENIS

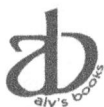

aly's books

www.alysbooks.com

Your book | Our mission

Aly's Books
PO Box 25
Kingsville Vic 3012
Australia
www.alysbooks.com

ISBN: 9780987529664

Catarina, Sue and Chris, Loretta, Anthony (Kouta),
George, Chris and Theresa Lindsay.
All my amazing family, friends, the people who pre-purchased
the first copies and everyone who has inspired, supported and stuck
with me throughout my life. I dedicate this to you.

Contents

Foreword

It's difficult to reflect my life through writing, especially when I'm only in my 30s and still have the rest of my life to look forward to. Over the years I have accumulated some terrific accomplishments and I've also had my fair share of emotional highs and lows.

Self-discovery, passion, loyalty, love, hate, friendship, compassion and dedication; those are just some words to describe this story. I could never have accomplished what I have in such a short amount of time without the love and support of some very inspirational people in my life.

As I take a look back through my life, I reflect on the past as a child, growing into a teenager, then an adolescent and then finally an adult. It's hard to talk about certain things that have happened in my life, but as I look back on all of it now, it's made me the stronger, happier person I finally am today.

This journey is about development, the development of my self-esteem, my inner self and most importantly, the development of who I am today and who I could be in the future.

My story tackles some of the toughest issues that I have gone through in my life. Many of these issues are faced by a number of people today; bullying, lack of confidence, self-image, obesity, self-control and acceptance of who we truly are.

It's not always about being tough or being popular. Sometimes it's about what's right in front of you and the people you are surrounded with. I learned from my own experiences that not everything is as it seems; far from it actually.

Recently I have gone through a major transformation and completely changed my lifestyle to accommodate this change. I was someone who always hated sport or any form of physical activity like running, exercising and stretching.

Although it has taken me a long time to get to where I am at this particular moment, I am still not where I want to be, and that's because my journey is far from over.

Not having people around me who I could ask for help was one of the hardest things I had to endure. If I have learnt anything in life, it's that life was never meant to be easy. However, the choices we make determine how we shape our destiny, in happiness and in adversity.

For many nights, I sat around feeling sorry for myself and feeding junk into my body because that was the way I dealt with emotion. Being bullied and picked on at school was challenging and all I did was sit around and let it go on because I lacked one thing: *confidence*.

Even as I got older, life got harder, and whenever it was tough I felt like giving up and many times I did. I would lock myself in my room for hours and cry myself to sleep because I felt sorry for myself. Self-pity would prove to be a destructive habit that I had to break if I was going to transform myself into a happier and healthier person.

I went through Primary School and most of Secondary School with hardly any friends. I tried to ignore the lack of social interaction, my feeling of isolation and awkwardness, but the hardest part wasn't ignoring it, but admitting it and confronting the fears that would inhibit my ability to form meaningful friendships.

I know there are many people out there who may be in this very situation. All I can say to you is, believe in yourself, face your fears and never abandon hope, because anything is possible.

I am not a nutritionist, a doctor or a psychologist, so I can't give you advice, but I can share with you, my experiences. I can share with you how I dealt with the situations and how I overcame the hurdles in my life and hope that in some way they can help you.

I was fortunate enough to meet some very special, inspirational and dedicated people in my life. Many who I hope will continue to be a part of my life in the future. Being surrounded by these people helped me through the tough times because they were all there to support me when I needed them the most. If you surround yourself with positive people, you will be inspired to see yourself in a positive light.

It's important for everyone to know how these people inspired me and yes, this is a story about me, but in many ways, these people are all a part of me.

I've changed my lifestyle and that has helped me enter a whole new world of writing, health, fitness, hard work and most importantly, I have discovered who I really am.

Be patient and follow me on this journey. A journey that has made me cry, laugh, be happy, but most of all, it's made me change my outlook on my life. It's given me strength, confidence, self-esteem and motivation to create and achieve goals I never thought possible.

I hope this journey is one that you will all love and enjoy reading as much as I have enjoyed living and writing it.

Steve

Chapter 1

Growing Pains
1981–1988

On April 10th, 1981, screaming down the walls of the maternity ward with my lungs at the Preston and Northcote Community Hospital, I graced the world with my presence. It was the early hours of Friday morning at 5am weighing just over 9lb.

During the early years of my life I grew up in Lalor, a suburb in Melbourne's north, in a modern 3 bedroom home which was situated directly across the road from my paternal grandparents' home. Growing up with European parents meant that my grandparents couldn't speak any English and so I learned to speak the traditional Macedonian language at a very young age.

Whilst Mum and Dad worked full-time I was left in the care of my grandparents until they returned home from work every evening. My grandparents, in their late 60s at the time, were not employed and stayed home looking after myself and my older cousin James, who lived in the same street.

In 1984, on Wednesday March 7th, I became an older brother to Paul, who also entered the world at the Preston And Northcote Community Hospital.

I remember my 4th birthday party at home, when my brother Paul was less than a month old. We had the extended family over for my birthday and also introduced everyone to the new arrival in the family.

Having a younger brother was a lot of fun, we got to play games together, grow up together, and we played together in the back yard. We jumped on the trampoline together, read each other stories and even rode our bikes together.

In January 1986 it was time for my cousin and I to attend our first day of school. I still lived across the road from my grandparents and my cousin was still down the street.

We attended a Catholic School only a 10 minute walk from home, so it was convenient for our grandmother to drop us off and pick us up each day. I remember wearing the dark green jumper and track suit pants with the red coloured skivvy underneath each day as we walked to school, hand in hand.

My cousin and I were never in the same class, but our classrooms were next to each other and we always played together in the playground during recess and lunch. We often spent a lot of time on the play equipment or running around on the oval. Other times we played ring a ring a rosy with the girls in our class.

The thing that I looked forward to the most at school was Fish & Chip days. Both of our teachers would dress up as little school girls with pig tails in their hair and they would order fish & chips for the class. It was fun to see the teachers behave like school girls. It made us feel more comfortable around them because they were at our level and we got to treat them like little girls rather than our teachers.

Our classrooms were next to each other and separated by a door on the inside which could be opened to join the two rooms together. When we had fish & chip days the teachers would open the doors so that the two classes were one and we all ate our fish & chips together. I enjoyed these days because we got to interact with the other classes and we got to have a lot of fun. It was a nice change to eat something different from the traditional sandwiches that Mum used to make me every day for school.

I remember one particular incident that happened in Grade 1, 1987. I had a toilet "accident" and my teacher had to give me a change of tracksuit pants to wear. When my cousin saw me he asked what happened. I couldn't really lie so I told him exactly what happened, but I made him promise not to say anything to our grandmother.

As soon as we got home that night and walked in the door my grandmother noticed that I was wearing different pants to the ones I had left with. She asked me what happened to my pants? I told her that we were playing a game at school and my pants got ripped and the teacher gave me these ones to wear.

My cousin couldn't control himself; he burst out laughing and told my grandmother what really happened. I kept trying to tell her that he was lying, but she believed him and not me. I was so embarrassed. I remember my cousin telling my grandmother "Steven did poo in his pants grandma and the teacher had to give him a new pair of pants."

Dad was a self-employed carpenter who worked with my uncle, my cousin's Dad, and they had their own business. In mid-1988, Dad's business started to prosper and in turn, he started to get more and more work on the Mornington Peninsula.

Most times, when Dad was working down at the Peninsula, he would be away for a week and come back on the weekends before travelling back again. This was putting strain on the family and Dad realised it was simply too hard to continue the way he was.

Half way through Grade 2, Dad decided that we would all move down to the Mornington Peninsula to a small seaside suburb known as Rye. I was taken out of my current school whilst Mum and Dad packed our things ready for the move.

I was 7 and Paul was just over 4 years old when we made the move down to Rye. When we arrived, Dad had bought a beautiful modern 3 bedroom home with a gravel drive-way, which was located on the corner of a busy main road and a quiet suburban street. On weekends, Dad usually took me to work with him to help him out. I hated it. Sometimes I used to hide in my room whenever Dad was looking for me so I could get out of going to work with him. The thing that I hated about working with Dad was that I found it boring and there was never anything fun for me to do there. As a kid I wanted to have fun, not be on a work site lifting timber or shovelling dirt around.

My uncle purchased a block of land about 10 minutes up the road from where we lived. He started building his own house whilst he was living in Lalor and would often come down on weekends to visit while he was working on his house.

After his divorce, my uncle also moved down to Rye to continue his work commitments with my Dad. Due to their demanding schedule, it was hard for either of them to have any free time and my uncle's house wasn't quite finished. As he was building his own house, my uncle lived in it the whole time through the building process. I never got to see James again for many years after that. Moving away from him was hard because we were so close and we had spent most of our childhood together. James moved away to live with his mother while my uncle moved to Rye and we lost all means of contact.

Chapter 2

After a few weeks we had finally settled down in Rye and I started at my new school. The school was located about a 25 minute walk from home. Mum used to walk me to school every day and then she would meet me at the gate after school.

As I had left school halfway through the year, I was going to pick up right where I left off. On my first day I was taken to my new classroom where I met my new teacher and class mates.

I was put into a class known as 1 & 2A. It was what we called a composite class when teachers taught two year levels at the same time in the one classroom. It was quite strange being in a classroom where there were kids my age, but also older than me as well. It took some time to adapt to the new environment. I started school half way through the year so I had a lot of help from my teacher and some of the other kids. Soon enough I started to make some new friends.

The following year in 1990, it was time for Paul to start his first day at school also. We were dressed in our summer shorts and t-shirts as we walked, hand in hand, down to school.

For the first few years, Mum walked Paul and I to school every day and then came to pick us up every night until we were both old enough to walk ourselves.

With our family now living in Rye and our relatives remaining back in Melbourne, our extended family started buying beach houses in Rye so they could come down and visit us on weekends.

Going through primary school wasn't easy. I was always a small porky kid, often hanging around with the girls and staying in the classrooms with all the teachers during recess. All the boys at school wanted to kick around a footy or play cricket. I never enjoyed sport so I preferred to stay inside with the girls and write on the blackboard or read books. I also didn't want to get into trouble by the teachers so I avoided hanging around with the boys for that reason.

I didn't make many male friends whilst in primary school; I didn't get along with them. I was never confident in myself at school and it showed with the boys. They always saw me as an easy target, someone they could pick on and push around.

I soon became a victim of childhood bullying; the boys started picking on me. I told my parents about them and even reported them to the teachers, but this just aggravated them even more. They continued to bully me, showing no signs of remorse at all.

Even after school, the bullying continued, the boys followed me on my way home, pushing me into the bushes, teasing me and calling me nasty names. They would yell out things 'Fatty boomba, Loser' or even worse 'A Wanka', all of which usually made me cry. It didn't help that I was slightly overweight either; I couldn't fight back and defend myself.

One afternoon, my maternal grandparents had come down to visit from Glen Waverley. They also had a beach house which was about a 5 minute drive away from our house. I had gone for a ride on my bike when I was approached by the 'bullies' from school once again.

They started teasing and bullying me, pushing me around and picking on me because I was fat and weak. They grabbed me by my arm and took me to the top of a hill where they tied me up to a tree with a rope and they dropped my pants down to my ankles. They left me there while they ran down the hill and let the air out of my tyres before walking off.

I was in tears, crying and holding my head down in shame. I remember my grandfather driving by in his Red Ford. He stopped by the side of that hill and looked up at me, almost in tears himself. He climbed out of the car, walked up to me and untied me from the tree and we walked down to the car together. I remember him taking me home and telling my Mum and grandmother what had happened. I was so ashamed and upset that I started to cry.

I was always called a 'Teacher's Pet', and rather than call me by first name, everyone called me 'Genis' or 'Genis the Menace'. I hated it. I had such low self-esteem and no confidence in myself due to my weight and image. As a result, I was always hanging around the teachers and their offices. Perhaps this is why boys hated me so much as opposed to the girls. The boys were always skinny and better looking than I was, which is probably why they enjoyed picking on me so much.

I hated exercise and P.E was my least favourite subject. I remember athletics days at school where we would go to a reserve in Rye. Out of all the sport activities that we did on those days, I dreaded the 500m sprint. Even during normal P.E classes at school, I would always fake an injury just so I could get out of doing the class. During these classes I was constantly out of breath and always coming last whenever we did any form of running exercises.

I recall our school's Blue Light Disco. I remember a guy called Dean, an evil, skinny looking thing. He was what you would call one of the 'tough guys' in primary school and he hated me. I recall him entering the hall where the disco was being held with another guy, wearing a singlet and jeans.

He walked right up to me and pulled me into a head lock and held me in that position. My weight and image was a reason I couldn't defend myself against this guy and I couldn't free myself from the headlock. I remember being in that position until security came in and broke us apart some time later. I remember telling Dean to let go of me, leave me alone and stop picking on me. Hearing me say this just gave him more ammunition to keep going as he thought that I was trying to be 'tough'.

I was also involved in the school choir and every Monday morning at assembly we would sing the school's theme song. Being in the choir, I was also involved in many of the school's singing and dancing productions. I loved to sing. I would always sing to the old records that Mum and Dad played at home. When there was the opportunity to be in the school choir, I jumped at the chance of singing and dressing up for productions. I always had a lot of fun with the other students when I went to these school events.

Sunday June 2nd 1991, the third and final Genis brother arrived. Christopher was born at the Rosebud hospital, and I was once again an older brother with an age gap of 10 years between us. A few days after Christopher came home from hospital, Mum and Dad sold our house and we moved down the road to our new home.

After four years in Rye, Dad started picking up work again in Melbourne and was once again travelling between Rye and Melbourne on alternate weeks, as he was when we were living in Melbourne. Dad purchased a block of land in Epping in Melbourne's outer north and started building our new family home. He was planning on moving back to Melbourne for work, this time on a permanent basis.

Halfway through the year, it was time to decide which High School I would be attending. Dad told me that although we would be moving back to Melbourne, it wouldn't be for at least another year. He decided, rather than start at a school in Rye and then transfer after a year, it was best that I move back to Melbourne on my own. I would live with my grandparents once again for a year until Dad finished his building commitments and then move to Melbourne with Mum, Paul and Christopher.

By the end of 1992 I was enrolled at my new High School in Epping and it was my Grade 6 graduation. All the Grade 6s proceeded to the Rye Civic Hall where we all sat down in our chairs. Our school principal walked onto the stage and proceeded to read out our names as we all walked onto the stage and collected our graduation certificates. I walked onto the stage and shook his hand as he handed me my certificate and said "all the best at your new school mate" as I walked off.

Chapter 3

High School: The Early Years
1993–1995

January 1993 was a scary time for me as I started my first year of High School. I was living with my grandparents while Dad, Mum, Paul and Christopher were still living in Rye. I very rarely got to see my Mum and Dad whilst I was living with my grandparents. They usually only came down once a fortnight for the weekend and then headed back to Rye again. Whenever they left, I always cried because I missed them so much. Even talking to them on the phone was cut short as long distance phone calls were very expensive. I couldn't really do much while I was living with my grandparents. I couldn't go out with my friends or go to the movies, mainly because I had no money and my grandparents were not working. It was also hard because I had to ask my grandparents' permission to go some-where and they didn't know what answer to give me because my parents had left me in their care. There were many times when I just couldn't cope staying with my grandparents. I had no one to talk to about it and I always missed my parents and my brothers.

I was 12 when I started High School and the classes were grouped into 4 different coloured units. They were Silver Unit, Gold Unit, Red Unit and Blue Unit. Blue Unit was for Years 11 & 12 while the others were purely for Years 7–10.

In Year 7, I was put into Silver Unit. My teachers seemed nice, as did the students. The first bell rang at 8:45am, prompting students to make their way to their lockers and get their books for class. The second bell rang at 8:55am for Home Group, which was where we got our names marked off the attendance roll for the day. The final bell then rang at 9:00am to commence first period.

On our first day we got our timetable, we had six periods a day, averaging 48 minutes each, with a 20 minute morning recess break and 50 minute lunch break. School finished at 3:06pm daily.

Some of the kids I went to school with were also of European background, many of whom were Macedonian.

I was getting settled into High School and getting used to all my classes, teachers and trying to make some friends. Things appeared to be going ok, until I started P.E.

I remember my first class, my P.E teacher was a relatively tall guy with an accent in his early 40s. At the age of 12 I couldn't really understand the difference between a crush and a fantasy. I was really attracted to my teacher, but my attraction towards him wasn't in a homosexual way. Having no confidence in myself and such low self-esteem I couldn't talk to anyone about the way I was feeling. The fact that this was my teacher as well, made the situation worse.

I was overweight and very uncomfortable with my image, and seeing my teacher with a fit healthy physique was what I was attracted to. I couldn't tell anyone how I felt when I myself didn't know how I really felt, or what others might think about the attraction. I guess I was more scared of being bullied or called a homo-sexual which is why I kept it to myself.

It was no secret that I hated sports and I remember this one partic-ular class we had. Our teacher made us do a fitness circuit known as the creek run. It was along a creek which had a running track along-side it. As you could imagine, being overweight and unfit, I came second last.

This one particular guy, Drew, was also overweight and was just as unfit as I was. I remember heading back to the gym after we fin-ished the run and our P.E teacher telling everyone out loud that we had all done a good job. Well, everyone except Drew and I, "because they are overweight", he told the class. I also remember him telling us that we could sit it out next time.

Initially, Drew and I made a joke about it and I remember him saying that he was proud to be overweight because it meant that he got out of doing the run in future classes. I guess I was happy about it at the time because it meant I didn't have to do the run either. Thankfully it was only compulsory to do P.E from Year 7 to Year 9.

It was tough going through Year 7. I tried so hard to make friends, male and female, but I couldn't; I just didn't seem to fit in. I had put on more weight since leaving Primary School. The problem I had, living with my grandparents during my first year of High School, was that my grandmother fed me traditional European food. With these meals I would also often have one to two slices of bread. I soon got into the habit of having three to four, sometimes even five slices of bread with my meals each night, adding more carbs to my body. Even though my grandparents knew that I was putting on weight, they didn't say anything. All they cared about was making sure that I was fed well.

Dad played a lot of soccer in his youth and he loved the sport; he started taking me to soccer matches on weekends. I remember this one time when I was 13, Dad enrolled me to play soccer for the local team. He knew how much I hated it, but he still enrolled me regardless. He thought it would help me to stay fit and learn to play a sport. I hated sport; I was never active and a bit lazy at times. I ignored my body and never thought there was a problem with the way I looked so I never did anything about it. For this reason, I never picked up a sport because I just did not have the motivation or the desire to do it.

Things appeared to be going really well for me in High School; I had settled down, learnt what to expect and met all of my teachers, and started to get used to all my subjects, then everything started again.

The boys in the class started to see that I was a real 'nerd' and a 'teacher's pet' and once again people started calling me 'Genis'.

All the boys in my class were the 'cool guys' and didn't want to be seen hanging around with a nerd so they all started to distance themselves from me. The guys were always skinnier than I was; they always played up in class rather than do any work. While I had my uniform nicely pressed and presentable, they always wore sloppy clothes. Even in the school yard, they were always swearing, using words like 'Shit' or 'Fuck', words that I was always too scared to use.

Once again, it was the girls who I surrounded myself with. Many of them were genuinely nice and caring, but the others, although they never said it, I knew, deep down, they just really felt sorry for me. I knew they felt sorry for me because they always had their own group of friends that they would always hang out with. Whenever they would see that I was sitting alone, they would always invite me to join their group, which were always girls.

As the year went on, things started to go from bad to worse, only now it wasn't just the boys being evil and nasty to me, the girls started too. It would start with whispering things under their breaths and then move on to things much worse like name calling. First it started with names like idiot or dickhead, and then it would lead to much worse names like poof or faggot. It eventually got to the point where I was afraid of going to school all together in fear of what would happen to me that day. I was scared of being called a faggot or a poof, mainly because I was confused with my sexual preference and actually did find myself attracted to many of the guys, some of which were in my classes. I was afraid that they might find out how I felt about them and start nasty stories or worse, beat me up.

I reported it to the teachers; many of them told me to ignore it. It was hard to ignore something like that, especially when I had classes with these people every single day. It eventually got to the point when at lunch times, I started staying indoors with all the teachers rather than go outside.

Most times I dreaded waiting outside a classroom in between classes. I was always scared of what people would say or do to me, knowing that I was most vulnerable when there were crowds around because I couldn't defend myself. By the end of Year 7 things had still not changed and I was really unhappy. I decided to talk to the teachers again and tell them that I wanted to change classes next year.

In 1994, Mum, Dad, Paul and Christopher moved down to Melbourne. We didn't yet have our own place so we lived with my Dad's parents for another year while Mum and Dad continued to work full-time.

When school resumed the following year I hadn't heard anything from my teachers about changing classes. I remember running late for school, and as I entered the building of Silver Unit, my teacher told me that we had Science and to go to the science room. I almost cried and remember telling her that I was no longer in her class. She said to me "yes you are, off you go".

I went to the science room and sat down; as the teacher read our names on the roll she called me to the front of the room. I remember her telling me that my transfer to another class had been accepted, but it appeared that I was still on her roll for some reason.

By the middle of that day, I moved to my new class in Gold Unit. I started to make some new friends and most of the students seemed nice.

In 1995 I was in Year 9 and just turned 14. I studied Drama as a subject at school. I loved acting; it was so much fun being on stage and getting into character, even if it was only for an hour.

The school had regularly put on Drama productions in the past where you could invite family and friends to come along and watch your performance. That year I was involved in the school production of *The Phantom of the Soap Opera* a mock of the musical *The Phantom of the Opera*. Although my part was short and gave me minimal stage time, it was so much fun being up there with all that make up and lights.

My character in the play was in love with a girl whose contract forbade her to date anyone else unless they worked on the same set as her. I have to admit it was a little intimidating at first as the student who played my love interest in real life was three years my senior.

We had lunch time rehearsals and sometimes late night after

school rehearsals as we prepared ourselves for the opening night in September. Our school was also chosen to participate in the local arts show held at a community centre in Preston. We only performed the first scene of our play, but it was in front of a large, sold out audience, in a huge auditorium. Both my grandparents, my aunty, uncle and my parents, who had front row seats, came to see me that night.

We finally performed the play in our school's drama room over three nights on a Wednesday, Thursday and Friday evening at 7:30pm. I recall one time during my performance when my character was supposed to be on stage; I was backstage changing into my costume and my shoe was in a double knot. I couldn't undo the knot and I had to be on stage. The other girl on stage was waiting for me, so I just went out with one shoe on and the other half off hoping no one would notice.

By the end of 1995, Mum and Dad had found a small place for us to live while Dad finished building our house in Epping. The place we rented was located right next door to my brother Christopher's kindergarten. Mum and Dad worked as factory hands for a company in Reservoir and Dad got me a casual job there over the Christmas school holiday period until I returned back to school. I did a lot of production work at that factory. The company made household cleaning products such as mops, brooms and sponges. The job required a lot of packaging work, packing the products into boxes and then stacking them onto pallets ready for shipment.

The work hours were from 7:30am to 4:00pm each day. I didn't enjoy the 6:00am wake ups every morning though, but the experience was great. I got to learn about the workforce and what it was really like to be working in that sort of environment. I didn't really get much of a chance to enjoy my Christmas School holidays, but while the other kids were out spending their money, I was earning mine.

Chapter 4

Adolescence
1996 – 1998

By the time I got to Year 10 in 1996 I was almost 15 years of age. I remember sitting in Home Group and the teacher was reading out a student newsletter. The student newsletter kept us up to date with events that were going on, both in and out of the school.

One morning, our Home Group teacher was reading the bulletin and there was an article about a major department store which was opening soon in a new shopping centre that they were building in Epping. The article stated that applicants needed to be 15 years of age or older before applying. I wasn't 15 until April that year so I couldn't apply.

Sometime in March I remember a student that I went to school with telling me that she had applied for a job at the new shopping centre. I was curious and asked her how; as the shopping centre wasn't due to open for another month. She told me that it was advertised in the local paper.

I recall reading the article that night when I got home; I put together a resume and planned to apply for the position. The following day, after school, I walked to the shopping centre and they had a small section open for people wishing to apply for jobs.

When I arrived I was introduced to the manager of the store and she handed me a job application form. I told her that I wasn't 15 yet, but she told me that the employment age was 14 and 9 months, this meant that I was old enough to apply.

The job I was applying for was a major supermarket as a service cashier, or what was known as a checkout operator back then. When I finished the application I handed it back to the manager with my resume and I was told I would hear from her in a few weeks. Every night after that, each time the phone rang, I thought it was the manager telling me I had got the job.

One night we were sitting at home when I received a letter in the mail from the job I had applied for. As I opened the letter and read through it, I realised that I was unsuccessful for the position at this stage. It was the first job I had ever applied for and I was really upset about it so I decided to call them for some feedback.

When I called, I spoke to the manager directly and she advised me that the letters were automatically generated and they were sent out to everyone. She informed me that I had, in fact, been successful for the position and I would be starting work during the April school holidays before the shop opened.

I was so happy, that feeling of joy running through my mind as I sat there and told Mum and Dad the news, they were both happy for me.

So on the April school holidays I went down to the shopping centre and made my way to the store. We were given a few shifts a week to train and prepare ourselves for the store's opening in less than two weeks.

In April 1996, I turned 15 and Epping Plaza opened its doors to the public and it was my first shift. I recall the chaos of crazy shoppers grabbing their opening special bargains that were on store wide. Dad had finally finished building our house just enough for us to move in, so we packed our bags and left our rental house.

That year at school, I chose to study Drama again. I had so much fun last year that I wanted to do it again. I was once again involved in the school's production. That year we did a production called *King Artie and the Knights of the Rad Table*, a mock of *King Arthur and the Knights Of The Round Table*.

I wasn't playing a lead role, but my role was slightly bigger than the previous year. This time around I actually played two different roles on stage. Unlike my first production, I had a lot more stage time in this play. I had actually made my own costumes and playing two roles, I was able to fool the audience with a wig and some crafty make-up. I loved the whole experience and I loved being up on that stage. I fell in love with Drama when I did it as a subject and I jumped at the chance to be a part of these productions. We (the other actors and I) got along really well on the night and supported each other. We helped each other with our lines before walking out on stage and in between scenes. We also helped one another get ready into our costumes.

The play was a great success, my parents and brothers came along to the production and they really enjoyed themselves. The fact that we all had fun, interacted together and didn't cause a panic was what made the whole show a complete success by all. I loved the whole experience and after it was over, I wanted to do it all over again.

In Year 10, students were also given the opportunity to do some paid work experience for 2 full weeks, at a rate of $5 per day, to prepare ourselves for the real working world when we left school. By the time I was in Year 10, my mind was pretty much made up and I wanted to be a teacher, so I decided to concentrate on that field when looking for my work experience opportunities.

I chose to do work experience at one of the local Primary Schools, teaching grades 5 & 6 for one week and then kindergarten students for the second week. It was fun being a teacher. I particularly enjoyed the primary school experience more, as the teacher let me get involved in teaching the class. The grade 5 & 6 teacher even let me teach one class on my own while she sat and supervised. It was a Maths class, I gave the kids a problem solving exercise and got to stand there and watch them all try and work it out for themselves. With the kindergarten it was more about interacting with the kids as opposed to actually teaching them. It was also great because it meant I could be with my baby brother Christopher all day. While I was working with the kindergarten kids, the teacher got me to play games with them, prepare their afternoon milk snacks, and also colour in with them. When the kids were outside we usually played in the sand pit and built sand castles or played on the play equipment.

By the year's end I was still working my job at the supermarket and over the Christmas holidays I went to work with Mum and Dad at the factory again.

By 1997 the reality of high school had officially sunk in. I was about to turn 16 and planned on having a party at home. The final two years of high school were known as VCE, (The Victorian Certificate of Education). In Year 11 and 12 we had the option of choosing our subjects other than English.

We did a total of 6 subjects in Year 11. I chose English, Biology, Further Maths, Accounting, Home Economics and Information Technology.

I turned 16 in April and to celebrate my sweet 16th, I had my birthday party at home. I guess it was also a house warming party as it was the first time many of the relatives had actually been to our home since we moved in. Dad finished working at the factory and went back to his building commitments full-time with my uncle.

I also started my first serious relationship that year, dating a girl called Whitney. Whitney was only 13 when we started dating and I was 16. To say that her father disapproved of our relationship is an understatement. His disapproval wasn't of me as a person or my age, it was more because I was European and she was Australian. Whitney was always telling me that her father preferred she dated Australian men, but Whitney ignored his wishes, telling him that she would date whoever the hell she wanted. He was never racist towards me and never spoke badly of me, but I could always sense the awkwardness whenever I walked into their home. I guess the age factor did play a small part in it as well even though he never truly admitted it. In the end he could see that I loved and respected his daughter despite my culture and my age. He could see that I was good to her and I always made her happy. In the end, he saw that I was a decent guy and accepted our relationship.

During Years 8–10, it appeared that things were going ok. I mean I still didn't have that many friends, but Whitney and I were together. Compared to what I was going through in previous years, it felt like my life was improving.

All that soon changed. In Year 11, I became the victim of bullying once again. This time it was much more serious, the words that were coming out of people's mouths were hurtful and disgusting. Soon I become a stranger in my own school. I couldn't walk to classes alone, in fear that someone would jump out and start pushing me around. The guys continued to call me 'poof' and 'faggot'; unfortunately, even as they got older, they never matured. The boys were always punching me on the arm as well, not to the extent of bruising me or anything like that, but it still hurt. People bullied each other because it made them feel good about themselves. When they were surrounded by their friends (and girls) that gave them an ego boost and they chose to punch me and call me these names as a way of making them look good.

Even in class, I found myself sitting next to the girls instead of the boys and usually in the front row. If I ever did sit next to one of the guys, it was because it was the only seat left in the classroom and I had no other option.

I guess I was lucky after school; many students caught the bus or lived in different directions to me, so the walk home was usually pretty safe. Over time it got worse, many of the boys teased me in class whenever the teachers left the room and most of the time the nasty girls joined in as well. Apparently, everyone thought it was fun to tease the nerdy kid in class and say spiteful things because it made them look big and tough. It was something I had to deal with every day and I just sat there and took it all. I was always the only one in class who got bullied or picked on. The students were smart however, they waited until the teacher would leave the classroom for a few minutes before they would yell out "Genis, did you fart?" or "What are you looking at Genis?" They wanted to embarrass me in front of the entire class. I always tried to keep my head down and hide the tears forming in my eyes. As soon as the teacher would walk back in, it was as if nothing had ever happened. I had gone through most of High School being bullied and although there was no physical abuse, the verbal abuse was much worse.

I was always going to the teachers after school or during recess and told them what was happening. The teachers never physically caught the students doing these things to me so they could never prove it; this made it hard for them to implement any form of punishment.

In April 1997, I got my Learners Permit. Dad had been saving all the money that I was earning from working at the factory and I had also been saving my own money from working at the supermarket. There was a guy that Dad was working with who was selling his car. A 1978 Yellow Holden Gemini, 5 speed manual. It wasn't the greatest car, but it was mine and I could practise my driving while I was on my Ls.

By April 1998 I was 17 and in my final year of high school. I was still on my Ls as I wasn't 18 for another year. The supermarket I worked for went into receivership and it was uncertain if any of us would keep our jobs, if and when the company was bought. Fortunately, the company was bought by another large supermarket chain, which is still operational today, and most of the staff kept their jobs.

Since I had been walking to and from school every day, and rarely ate during the day, I kept a good physique. I was working part-time and was constantly on the move, this helped me stay fit, healthy and active. As I look back at my 1998 Year 12 photo sitting in the front row, I can see that I was much thinner and healthier looking. Although I wasn't a very tall kid, my body was in the best shape it had been in for a long time.

At the end of 1998, Year 12 finished. I remember that night

in November, our Year 12 formal was at Greenville Receptions in Thomastown. A group of girls and I had all put in money to hire a limousine. It was our night, and I had never been to a school formal before, and was really looking forward to some fun and entertainment. I had bought a new dark green suit and a pair of black dress shoes. We stepped out of the limo and the girls and I walked into the reception, hand in hand.

We all sat at the same table and some of the teachers who were invited sat at the table opposite us. We had a three course meal and for the entertainment there was a DJ, who played the latest top 40 tracks. Most of us were still under the age of 18 so there was no alcohol at the event; we were only served water and soft drinks.

Everyone put all their differences aside on that night and we all enjoyed ourselves. Not surprising, most of the guys who were bullying me throughout High School, didn't come. I guess they thought they were 'too cool' to be there. As the night progressed, and we all got to interact with each other, we came to realise that some of us may not see each other again after High School.

At the end of the night we had no way of getting home as we had only booked the limousine to get us to the reception. I discussed with the girls what we could do and they suggested a taxi. I had never been in a taxi and after hearing stories about them on the news, I was actually quite scared to ride in one. Nevertheless, I jumped into the taxi with the girls as it drove us home one by one. I was the last one to be dropped off and made it home safely.

After that night, the reality of study and exams had officially settled in. Our first English exam on Friday October 30, 1998 was three hours of reading and writing and quite possibly the toughest test I ever took. What made it so hard was the fact that the English texts we were studying were very complex. I didn't understand the novels and throughout the year I was finding it hard to study. When it came to the exams I couldn't answer the questions because I hadn't understood the novels. Even after reading the exam for 15 minutes prior to sitting it didn't help me.

At the end of exams, it was finally time to celebrate and rejoice the end of high school. We had our annual 'dress up day' where we could dress up in anything we liked as part of our last day of year 12. I dressed up in a 'Scream' outfit which was a long black cloak with a white Ghost Face mask. Other characters ranged from Xena, Supergirl and even Scarlett O'Hara from *Gone with the Wind*. After dress up day we had our traditional "muck up day" where we could do whatever we wanted to the school, teachers and students, within reason, without getting into trouble. We were able to wrap toilet paper around buildings and throw flour and eggs at each other. The thing that everyone was looking most forward to was throwing egg and flour at the Vice Principal which had been a tradition at the school for many years.

I remember attending my first football match that year, Carlton vs. Essendon, at the Melbourne Cricket Ground with a friend of mine.

After two years, Whitney and I were still together and her father had finally accepted our relationship. In December that year, a massive blockbuster *Titanic* was released in cinemas. Whitney and I went to see the movie, in excess of 20 times in the cinema, during its entire theatrical run from December 1998 to June 1999. It's funny when you think about it, but I guess you can kind of say that we both contributed to the film's financial success in a way. Whitney and I never really knew too much about the story of the *Titanic*. All we knew was that it was a ship that sank, but we never knew the whole story. We didn't know what really happened and the huge amount of lives that were lost. We never studied it in school or read up on it either. The thing that drew us the most to the movie *Titanic*, aside from the disaster itself, was the fictional love story. It was the story about two completely different people from two completely different worlds who met and fell in love. That was Whitney and I all over, that was why we could relate to the movie so well and why we saw it as many times as we did.

Chapter 5

Young Adulthood
1999–2001

My life changed after school. I maintained my job at the supermarket and as I approached young adulthood, I got my driver's license and was still in a relationship with Whitney.

I also enrolled in a computer course at the local Northern Melbourne Institute of Tafe Campus in Epping. At the time the course seemed interesting and I enjoyed it for a short period. I only did it for six months and soon found it boring so I quit. Afterwards I started working for the supermarket full-time as well as various casual jobs with fast food giants and still worked at my Mum's factory from time to time.

One of the hardest things I had to deal with that year was a crazy fear that I had. I had heard on the news about all the wars going on overseas and the impact it was having on Australia. I had also heard about predictions that the world was coming to an end in the year 2000.

My biggest fear in life is death. I've always feared it from the moment I turned 18 and started reading about all these predictions. People always told me I was crazy and stupid and if it was going to happen then there was nothing I could do to control it. But I was too scared to accept that, and soon this fear about the world ending became an obsession.

Over time, my obsession became worse and I became more and more worried that one day it would happen and I would never wake up.

Everyone kept telling me that it was very unlikely that an event like that would ever happen in my lifetime. The disturbing thing was, during that year, there were two movies released six months apart about the end of the world. I guess now it was all just a crazy coincidence? The thing that scared me the most about these movies was, although they were not true stories, they were based on what could happen if an event like that really happened in our lives. I was so scared that I would live through it the way it was depicted in the movies.

It took me a while to really get over the fear and realise that I was over reacting and nothing was going to happen.

Everything soon changed in January 2001. I resigned from my position at the supermarket to pursue other career paths. It was at this point in my life where things started to take a negative turn. Being over 20, I now had my driver's license. I had a brand new car and so the luxury of having my own car meant that I drove everywhere rather than walk. Even a trip to the local Milk Bar, which was a ten minute walk from home, was avoided because I chose to drive there rather than walk.

I started to neglect my body and started feeding myself with junk. Soon the comfort of driving took over everything and it was from this point that I became lazy and less active and relied on my car for almost everything. I began to notice a serious change in my body and my image. The fact that I had my driver's license meant that I was spending more time in the car than on my feet.

Finishing work after midnight most nights meant that I couldn't be bothered waiting until I got home to prepare a meal and eat 'healthy.' Instead, a trip to the local fast food outlet seemed more convenient. The convenience soon became a habit, a dangerous habit of five to six times a week in fact, and late at night when the body is usually in wind down or sleep mode and unable to burn calories.

At the age of 20 I was still with Whitney who was now 17. On the morning of September 11th, 2001 I woke up and drove to Whitney's house to take her to school as I did every morning that year. When I arrived, Whitney was in the bathroom getting ready, when she asked me if I'd heard what had happened on the news. I didn't know what she was talking about and I looked at her with a perplexed expression.

She looked at me and said that two planes had crashed into the World Trade Centre. Initially I thought she was talking about the World Trade Centre in Melbourne, which was the other name given to the Crown Casino. When she said that planes had crashed, I also thought she meant as an accident.

It wasn't until Whitney and I watched the news that day and saw the nightmare unfold on the television that I realised the gravity of the event. I remember being speechless and all of a sudden my fears about war and the end of the world came flooding back.

Whitney looked at me and asked if I was ok. All the years that she had known me, she never saw me react like this before. I froze and didn't move until Whitney grabbed me by the arm and told me that she had to get to school. In the car, on the way to school, I explained to Whitney my whole fear about the end of the world. I had never told her how I really felt about it after all these years. Although Whitney was three years younger than me, she reacted more rationally and was more mature about it than I was. My irrational behaviour started to take a toll on our relationship. Whitney and I loved each other too much to let something like this ruin our relationship. She kept trying to convince me that it would never happen. For so long I had let my fears about the end of the world take over my life that I refused to believe anything Whitney was saying to me.

As the years went on I changed jobs several times and had various roles in various industries. I worked for a major utility company where I remained for two to three years from 2003–2005. This job unfortunately involved sitting at a desk answering phones for 6–8 hours a day and with no physical activity, it wasn't doing much for my physique. Over the years I got lazy and I started to put on quite a bit of weight. I was always sitting down at my desk. After working long hours, by the end of the day, I was always too tired to go for walks or go to the gym. My colleagues would start to see that I was putting on weight and as they started asking me questions about it, I began to ignore the issue. The more they spoke to me about it, the more I started to get angry and started eating as a way of punishing myself.

Chapter 6

In April 2002, I turned 21 and Paul was 18. Given that our birthdays were only a month apart we decided to have a joint 18th and 21st birthday party at home. Whitney and I had broken up, but we remained great friends and she attended my party that night.

In late 2002, a then unknown Australian female recording artist, Delta Goodrem, released a brand new single. The single premiered on a popular Australian Soap *Neighbours*, that she was starring in at the time. I remember watching the episode of the soap; in that episode she performed her single live on the show. The song was titled: *Born To Try* and it left a lasting impression on my life.

> *Doing everything that I believe in,*
> *Going by the rules that I've been taught,*
> *More understanding of what's around me,*
> *And protected from the walls of love,*
> *All that you see is me,*
> *And all I truly believe,*
> *That I was Born to Try*

After hearing the song on the show, the following day I bought the single. I studied and analysed the lyrics by heart, learning what the song was all about and what the lyrics actually meant. This song was about a road to discovery, it was about life, and making choices that may be right or wrong.

> *But you've got to make choices,*
> *Be wrong or right*

I don't know what happened or what triggered me to do what I did next, but I can say that it was perhaps the best decision I made that year. Day after day, night after night I played that song over and over again. I listened to it in the car everyday on repeat until I started imagining and visualising telling a similar story about me and my life.

By the time I was 22, I knew that I didn't want to spend all my life answering phones. I knew I could do better than that. After listening to that CD again, I enrolled myself into a local singing school. I remember walking into the building for the first time. I was nervous, excited and maybe even a little scared. I met the owner and I discussed with her what it was that made me want to join her school and what future I wanted for myself.

The following week on Saturday, I started my first 1 hour singing lesson with my teacher Courtney. By the end of the session I was very excited and determined to continue. Having already paid for five weeks in advance, I was very committed. When I got home that night, I looked in the mirror and looked at what was staring in front of me; a very unhealthy, unfit and unhappy person. That's when the reality finally sunk in; if I was ever going to have a chance at being a performer and being in the public eye, I had to do something about my image and very quickly.

The following day I made a choice, I started a very strict diet. A dear friend of mine, Kathleen, also wanted to do something about her image because she was just as unhappy as I was. We decided that we would do it together, using each other as inspiration and motivation.

A brand new well-known gym opened down the road from where I lived. Kathleen and I decided to go to the gym and see what membership deals they had. We spoke with one of the employees at the gym and indicated that although we were looking at losing weight and getting fit and healthy, we really couldn't afford an expensive gym membership. We were unsure how often we would actually be using the gym and its facilities.

The employee of the gym gave us some options to suit our financial needs, which would allow us to use the gym and its facilities. A standard monthly membership was $59.95 a month. I simply could not afford that, especially if I would only be using the gym one to two times a week.

As the gym had only just opened, they were looking at ways to get people interested to sign up and they didn't want to lose Kathleen and I as clients due to financial hardship. The employee signed us both up to an introductory membership known as "night owls" for only $19.95 a month; half of the original asking price.

The gym operated from 6am to 10pm Monday to Friday and this

membership would give us access to the gym, but only between the hours of 8pm to 10pm. If we used the gym outside those hours we just needed to pay an additional charge of $2 each time.

Kathleen and I thought it was a great idea and we decided to give it a try. Each night after work at around 7:45pm, we would meet up outside the gym and wait until 8:00. We took this one particular class, cycle, which was from 8–9pm every Tuesday. After finishing the cycle class we would do half an hour of weight training. We continued with this routine for several months every night. Within a matter of weeks, we both started to see the changes to our bodies and we started to feel good.

I continued with singing lessons every Saturday and because I was now starting to lose weight, this gave me the motivation to succeed with my music. I increased my lessons to two sessions per week, on Tuesday nights and Saturday mornings, as well as continuing to train at the gym with Kathleen.

At work, I remember talking to a colleague of mine, Sophie. Sophie told me that she had a Personal Trainer who trained her at the same local gym where I attended. Sophie spoke to her Personal Trainer, Josh, and explained to him that I was looking at starting personal training to lose weight and become healthy. She asked if he would consider taking me on as a client.

The next day at work, Sophie told me that Josh was happy to take me on as a client and gave me his number to schedule our first appointment. I called Josh after I finished work and we met up that night to discuss my fitness program. I started training with Josh three times a week for one hour sessions, either before or after work. As my results started to get more and more impressive, Kathleen and I looked at other ways we could increase our fitness and get into shape a lot faster. We came up with the idea to go for walks on Sunday evenings as we were both home and had no other commitments.

We both lived in Epping so this made it easier for us. Each Sunday night, I would leave my house at 7:00pm and drive to my friend's house. She lived less than 2 kilometres down the road. We planned our journey and proceeded to leave at 7:30pm.

Our walks consisted of an 8km round route, starting from her home and circling Epping before returning back to her home. When we first started the route, we were averaging approx. 1.5 hours to do the complete circuit. We stuck to the same route and each week we timed ourselves; our aim was to always decrease the amount of time it took us to walk the same route. From 1.5 hours we eventually got it down to 45 minutes within a few weeks, and then even 40 minutes towards the end; less than half the time when we started.

As time went on, Kathleen and I started to get into great shape. For six months I stuck with my regular personal training sessions with Josh at the gym, as well as our regular Sunday night walks whilst still continuing my singing lessons on Saturday mornings.

No more late night trips to fast food outlets, completely cutting out junk food and carbs and constant hard work and dedication for six months, saw me drop from approximately 110kgs down to 85kgs and maintain the weight.

After losing all the weight, I started to get my confidence back and began to feel good about myself again. I decided to put my new attitude to use. After almost a year of singing lessons, I had written a song. *Dreaming of You* was the name of my single. The song was about two very special girls in my life at the time, Whitney and Kathleen. I spent nine hours in a studio in Collingwood recording the single and then sent it off to be duplicated onto CD.

With my new look and image I asked a colleague of mine, Rose, to do a photo shoot for the CD cover as she was a photographer.

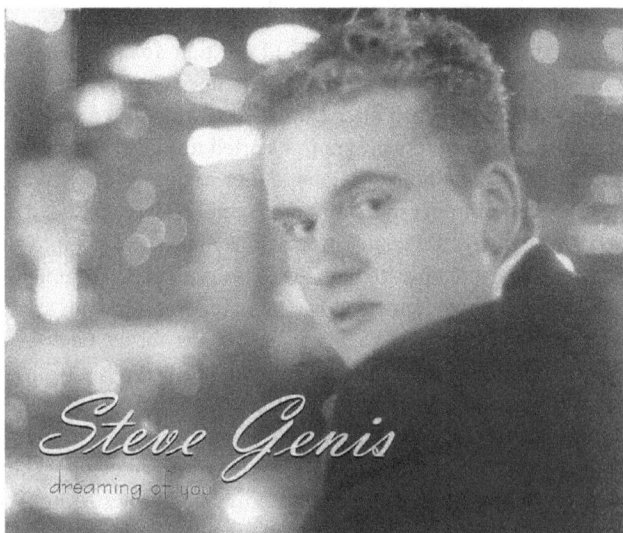

The CD single cover for *Dreaming of You* in 2003, I dropped to 85kgs, a loss of 25kgs, and my biggest and best achievement at that time.

I looked and felt great for the first time since I had left high school back in 1998. I was back under 100kgs and I loved the results that I had achieved. I was able to fit into nice thin pants again rather than baggy ones, and rather than look like a balloon every time I wore a suit, I actually looked good.

I made 500 copies of that single and invited my family and friends to a CD launch that I had to promote the song. I performed the song live on stage and although the turn out wasn't great, I had a great time and everyone enjoyed the song.

But I'm Dreaming of You,
But I know it's not true,
That I'll fall in love with you,
You're my strength, you're my rock,
You're the one I think of,
I can't see us to be in love,
I'm Dreaming of You.

Everyone that attended the launch loved the song. They loved my performance and most of all, they loved the lyrics. I was expressing myself through a song, talking about two loves and not being able to be with either of them. One was my best friend and the other was my lover.

Chapter 7

Lost and Confused

After a promising period in 2002–03 the next few years were difficult and perhaps some of the hardest ones I have had to endure. By 2004 my financial situation started to take a toll on me. With the constant stress in my life with family, work and my personal life, I started to lose motivation.

At 23 I pretty much had nothing, I still had a full-time job and I still had my car, but I had no money or savings. I was also single and didn't have anyone in my life.

At that time in my life I was constantly surrounded by negativity and had no self-esteem, or any confidence. It was difficult for me to confide in anyone, not my family or my friends, and I was going through something that I couldn't tell anyone about. I was worried that people would turn their backs on me and judge me.

I found myself being more and more attracted to males, but at the same time, I was still very attracted to girls. I was confused and didn't know which direction I wanted to go. Whenever I would see a really good looking male on the streets, I would just stare and be infatuated with him. When it came to girls, I found myself doing the same thing.

I fantasised about being with males, but in reality, I was too scared to act on my impulse and instead ignored my urges. I never acted on the way I felt and never told anyone about it. I know that people had their suspicions, and some people even confronted me about my sexuality, but I always told them I was straight.

I was more worried about what my family might think and I wasn't just talking about Mum and Dad. To be honest, I don't think I knew at the time exactly what I was feeling. I was lost and confused. Whitney was the longest relationship I had been in and at the time, when we broke up, even she thought it was because I was gay. I don't know why, but when Whitney and I broke up, it didn't affect me as much as it affected her. I stopped loving her, but it wasn't because I was drawn to males, I had just grown out of loving her. I felt that to continue on with the relationship, I would just be leading Whitney on and it wasn't fair on her. It was very hard going through that part of my life, not knowing how I felt and no one to talk to about it.

Even at work, I found myself attracted to many of my male

colleagues. I knew that it would be dangerous to ever let my feelings show or even look at them inappropriately, especially when most of these men were straight and married.

My urges got even harder to deal with, especially when I was hanging around the local shopping centre. There was this one particular guy who worked in one of the shops. I always found some excuse to go to his shop just so that I could stand there and stare at him. I never made it obvious, but whenever the moment started to get awkward and I couldn't stop staring, I left. Whenever I saw an attractive looking girl, I never knew how to react around one.

As a result of how I was feeling, I avoided the gym. I didn't want to be standing there looking at all the young, fit, athletic guys when I didn't have the perfect body. Josh also increased his fees and suddenly personal training became very expensive and I could no longer afford the sessions. Even cutting down to two sessions a week still wasn't financially affordable.

After almost a year of training, I could no longer afford it and I made the decision to quit altogether as there was no other option. As the popularity of the gym grew, more and more people were signing up and the gym eventually got rid of the 'night owl' membership; I was forced to sign up to a higher membership plan of $59.95 a month which I could not afford. Everyone increases their fees, I realise that, so I just used that as an excuse to take the easy way out of doing exercise.

A few weeks later I also lost my job with the utility company. I slowly started to put weight back on as a result of all the stress and anxiety that I was feeling. The only thing that kept me happy was going to the shopping centre and spending more and more time at that shop looking at the guy. He was roughly in his late 20s and there was something about him that I was attracted to. He was a great looking guy; he was young and dressed really well in designer clothes. This, and his well-built physique, was what attracted me to him the most. Even though I was overweight and unhappy with my image, I avoided doing anything about it because I lacked one thing, motivation.

It was hard to try and control my urges when all I kept doing was fantasising. I was using my urges as my comfort to ignore the issue of what was happening around me and avoid what I was doing to my body. Whenever I was in public with my friends, I tried so hard to control myself, but fighting the urge was not always easy.

Keeping this to myself was hard, but I was scared of people

judging me. My biggest fear wasn't being judged, it was being called a fag. That's the main reason why I didn't tell anyone, I couldn't handle being called a homosexual. I was too scared to tell my parents, especially my Dad, coming from a European background. I couldn't face his reaction, his disappointment and most of all, his disapproval.

Having no job, things started to look grim and financially I was struggling. With bills to pay, the stress was now reflecting on my weight and image more acutely. I continued with my singing; at the time it was the only thing that kept me motivated to keep on going and I went on to write some more songs. One of the songs that I had written was a song about my father. The song spoke about the dark times I had with my Dad and constantly walking into dead ends. It talked about not wanting to lie anymore about who I was; someone who was unhappy.

> *"I've been walking into dead end streets,*
> *Never knowing till now where I'm at,*
> *Somehow a voice kept telling me 'no' "*

> *"I don't want to lie anymore,*
> *Just want to be myself and not have to cry anymore,*
> *Just like a little boy, who falls off his swing,*
> *Once it's over, he forgets everything,*
> *Rub the dirt off my hands and tell me I'll feel better again*
> *I don't want to lie anymore"*

In mid-2004 I was faced with one of the hardest decisions that I had to make. I was now only working part-time and not earning a great deal of money. I was trying to hide from reality and what was happening to me, and I didn't want to accept what was happening around me.

In six months I had put on all the weight I had originally lost. I lost all hope and motivation and went back to my old ways; binging, eating junk and feeling sorry for myself. I was avoiding the reality, and the reality was that no one was going to pay money to watch a 'fat' person sing and dance. I threw away my dream of singing and being a performer and I quit singing after one year.

All I kept thinking to myself was that I was never going to meet anyone and fall in love so I may as well give up. Even though I wasn't sure about my sexuality, sometimes I was drawn to the thought of being with a guy. However, just as quickly as I thought of being with a guy, I took the idea out of my head. I let it go on for too long and soon the infatuations started to take control.

It was hard to admit to anyone back then that I was confused; I even had a tough time admitting it to myself. Although I don't regret the way that I felt, I regret never telling anyone how I felt. I was scared that I would be judged, unhappy and alone the rest of my life.

Chapter 8

Friendship

Throughout my life, I have met some amazing and inspirational people who have always been there to support and guide me. The biggest struggle for me wasn't always just my weight, image and self-esteem; it was also trying to meet new people and make new friends.

Back in 1998, when I was still working at the supermarket, I was working with a girl called Sam. We became very close friends and we spent a lot of time together outside of work. Sam introduced me to her family and some of her friends, one in particular was a guy called Chris Lindsay.

Chris was a tall, skinny guy, and he had the longest hair that I have ever seen on a guy. I remember the first time I met Chris, we were in Sam's house and Chris came over one night. Sam explained to me how she met Chris or 'CC' as he was better known back then. I recall the conversation when I asked Chris how he got his nickname. He told me that as he was growing up, Chris had a love for music and was always playing on his guitar, with his long hair and his physique, Chris resembled C.C. DeVille, the lead guitarist from the band *Poison*.

I have known Chris for just over fifteen years and I now consider him a close member of my family. At some point during 2004–2005 I had lost all contact with Chris. I had lost his number and hadn't seen or heard from him. One day, I was with my Mum walking through the shopping centre when all of a sudden I saw Chris, who yelled out "Steven" as he approached me pushing a pram with his then eight month old step son, Jayden.

The first thing Chris noticed about me was the amount of weight that I had actually lost since the last time he had seen me. Chris then introduced me to his then girlfriend, Theresa Frawley, who is Jayden's mother. As I was with Mum at the time, I didn't have much time to talk with Chris. We exchanged phone numbers again and agreed to catch up.

The years following, were let's just say, an adventure, a discovery of who I really was and what I had become. As the years went on, Theresa and I also grew very close. Sometimes, Theresa knew me better than I knew myself. She always knew whenever there was something on my mind and she always seemed to get it out of me. At one point, Theresa could see that I was struggling with my weight and that it had become an issue. Theresa was never one to criticise, but she always told me "rather than bitch about it, do something about it."

In November 2007, Chris and Theresa were married and I had the honour of being a groomsman at their wedding. The more that Theresa got to know me, the more she discovered about my past. She started to become more like a sister that I never had and I soon found myself telling her everything.

I remember being at their home one night and telling them both that I wasn't sure about my sexuality. It came as no surprise to either of them as they had suspected it for a few years, but never said anything about it. Theresa knew that this, as well as my weight, was obviously something that was affecting my self-esteem and my confidence and she came up with a way to get my confidence back.

We set out on a mission to do it together; Theresa wanted to help me on my journey. She came up with the idea that we could both go on evening walks, similar to what Kathleen and I had done a few years prior. It was never about Theresa needing to lose weight; it was about having her there for the support and motivation that I needed in my life.

So once a week, I would drive to Theresa's house in South Morang in the evenings and the two of us would go for our walk together.

The walk averaged about 8kms round trip and it would take us approximately 1 hour from the time we left her house to the time that we returned. We even attended regular aerobics classes at a local gym at 8am on Saturdays. This showed the determination and dedication that Theresa had towards me to help me on my road to weight loss.

We still remain in each other's lives and we now all consider ourselves family. As I look back through all these years and all the things that we have shared together, I will never forget all the times that Chris and Theresa were there for me. Having both of them, and their children, in my life has taught me to be a better person.

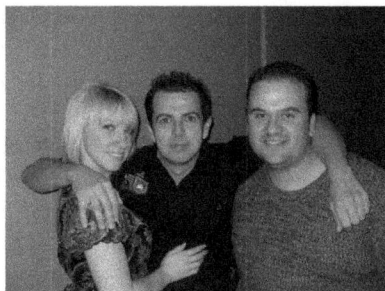

Dearest friends, Theresa Lindsay, Chris Lindsay and me in 2008.

Back in 2003–2004 when I was doing my singing lessons, dieting and personal training, I had come up with the idea of putting on my own stage production. It was a modern day re-telling of Shakespeare's most famous play *Romeo and Juliet*. I called my version *Romeo and Juliet: An Adaptation*, and I was looking for some actors to be a part of the production. I was telling Chris and Theresa (Lindsay) about it, and I remember Theresa telling me she had a close friend, who had actually done some professional acting work and she was happy to ask her to come along to audition.

At that moment, Jason Guthrie and Rebecca Lever (they were not married at the time) came into my life. Rebecca and Jason came along to one of the auditions that I was holding for the show and had a read through the script. Rebecca and Jason were happy with the script and decided to come on board and be a part of the production.

Unfortunately, after five or six months of weekly rehearsals, due to my poor management, lack of organisation and financial stress I cancelled the entire production. The worst part about it all was that I cancelled the show just two days before opening night when most of the tickets had already been sold. The cast had already told family and friends that they were involved in this upcoming show and most of them were really angry. I hurt many people as a result of my actions that day, most of them, including Jason and Rebecca, vowed never to speak to me again.

Along with everything else that was going on in my life at the time, I found it very hard to focus on anything positive. I hurt so many people and I started to punish myself. I started bad eating habits again, started feeling sorry for myself and started losing all the people around me as a result of all the hurt that I had caused. Again, I was turning to my urges and fantasies to make myself feel better.

True loyalty, friendship and forgiveness have played an important role in my life and helped me discover who I really was. The way I handled this production taught me valuable life lessons about what priorities are most important.

Although it took a few years, Jason and Rebecca eventually forgave me for what I did and I am extremely proud to have these two amazing friends in my life. It was their forgiveness that inspired me to go on; they both had every right to push me out of their lives and never speak to me again but instead, they forgave me.

Rebecca and Jason have both acknowledged my success and they continue to compliment and praise me for what I have achieved thus far. My life, by far, has been by no means easy, and there have been times where I have totally lost it and almost given up.

One particular time, in late March 2013, I was having a really bad day and I almost threw it all in because of a minor mishap that occurred with my regular training measurements. I posted my frustration on Facebook and within almost thirty seconds I had all my friends commenting.

I remember that day, Rebecca posted something on my wall that, and to this day, it is one of many inspirational comments that have stayed with me. It's a great example of the kind of inspiration that she has been to me. In response to my status that day Rebecca posted:

> *The hardest journeys are always the most rewarding.*
> *You have come so far and achieved so much, remember*
> *that when things get tough.*

She nailed it. All I needed that day was a little motivation to get me through that tough time and move on. Motivation has played an important role in my life. Whenever I lost the motivation to go on, that's when I turned to my friends to help me get through it all.

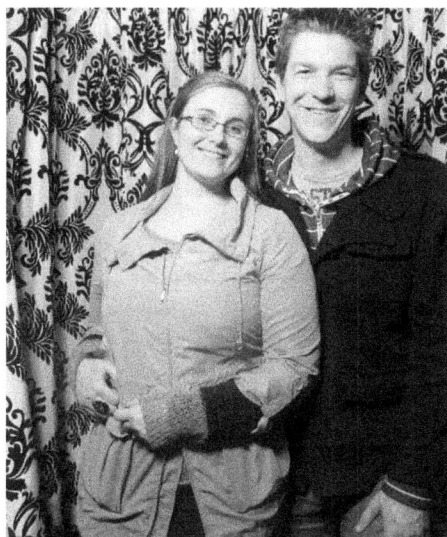

Jason and Rebecca Guthrie

I have had the honor of meeting some amazing friends in my life. Without the love and support of these people, I can say that I would have given up many times, but they have always been there to lift my spirits and put me back in my place, and not allow me to give up. Working at Village Cinemas, I was fortunate enough to meet many inspirational people. Two in particular have had a special part in my life during my time working with them; Kim Dellevergin and Hayley Griffiths.

I worked with both of these girls for two years at Village. Although they have only been in my life for a few short years, they continue, to this day, to be more than just my dear friends, they are also incredible role models.

Hayley Griffiths has always been one that has taken health and fitness seriously. Hayley has always participated in fitness activities such as boot camp. Up until recently, I can say that it's been hard for me to appreciate the true concept of health, fitness and sport, but with a new change of lifestyle and a different outlook on the future, all that has now changed.

Hayley always made fitness sound like a fun hobby rather than a painful exercise. She is a relatively tall girl who is very active and trim. I've met a lot of girls her age who are more interested in their boyfriends and going out partying, but Hayley has always taken her fitness seriously. Working with somebody like that every day has made it easy for me to stay motivated and focused, to lose weight and have a positive outlook on life.

Throughout the time that I have known Hayley, I have always been able to approach her confidently and openly talk to her about my weight and image and certain personal issues, without having to worry about what she would say or think. From the outset, Hayley has been there through my transformation and she has constantly complimented me on my success. I remember always telling Hayley how badly I had struggled to succeed and the first thing that I can recall Hayley telling me was: "Steve you should try boot camp".

Boot camp, was she serious? No chance, I hated exercise and the thought of boot camp made me sick and nauseous, all that exercise, sweating and not to mention all that fat flab bouncing around? No thanks. As proud as I am of my success, I think back to that conversation today and I can only imagine what my body would look like today if I had made the decision to start boot camp back then.

Every day I would walk into work on shifts that I was working with Hayley and I would look up at her and think to myself that maybe one day, I could be as fit and athletic as her and maybe, I should ask her what she does to keep herself fit. Hayley plays netball, so playing a sport and being active would give her the physique that she has and it would help her maintain it. Other than a little soccer, I hadn't played any form of sport.

Hayley is never one to complain about the pain endured during fitness, and in the years that I have known her, she is always speaking about it with a passion and how much she loves it. In recent years, Hayley's continuous support and kind words have kept me motivated throughout this journey. Walking into work every shift and hearing compliments out of Hayley is all the inspiration that I need to continue on my journey.

In late 2012, Hayley travelled to the U.S and returned just after the New Year in 2013. I remember her first shift back; we were both working in Gold Class together and by that stage I had lost about 15kgs and it was starting to show everywhere; my face, my chest and most noticeably, my stomach.

I remember the first thing that Hayley said to me as soon as I walked into the room: "Steve, you look amazing." I hadn't been complimented in such a long time and I didn't know how to react whenever I heard a positive comment, but I do remember being really happy, and it was a feeling that I had not had in a very long time. It made me realise how proud I was of my success because I knew that people had finally started to notice a change in my body and the way I looked and that was the best feeling.

Hayley continues to be an amazing inspiration throughout my journey and she is a dear and loyal friend. I am very grateful and honoured to have the privilege to work with her and share my success with her.

Kim Dellevergin or 'Kimmy D', as we all call her at work, is another great role model. No matter what mood I was in or how bad a day I was having, Kim could always make me laugh with her antics.

Kim is a very strong believer in health and fitness, much like Hayley, and Kim has also been there with me from day one of my weight loss journey. Kim has watched me try all the 'other diets' that haven't worked, and she always manages to see the comical side to it when I seemed to always let it get to me. Kim always came into work in a great mood, she never let a 'bad day' interfere with her work. Kim and I were huge fans of the movie *Burlesque* and quite often we would share some funny quotes from the movie. One particular quote was "Show a little more" which Kim and I often joked about whenever we would be on shift together. Kim often used this quote whenever she noticed a massive loss in my weight. She would come up to me and sing "Steve, show a little more, show a little less" and she would always put on a perfect American accent to get into character. Kim has also struggled with her image but, unlike me, she never let it affect her. I have always been able to open up to Kim just like I have with Hayley and sometimes on an even more personal and emotional level.

Every shift that Kim and I worked together she was always trying some diet. I don't really know why, as I never thought that she had a problem with her image, but we all look at our own bodies differently compared to others. During the time that I have known her, Kim has been an awesome inspiration in my life, especially through my weight loss over the last few months. She has inspired me to take on this journey because of her constant support. From day one Kim has never given up on me, even when my diets failed, she always seemed to come up with ways to make it feel a whole lot better without making me quit.

The most enjoyable thing that I love about Kim is watching and waiting to see what salads she is going to bring into work for dinner and then getting creative with them by adding Tuna.

Our dinners in the staff room would usually turn into a health session. Kim would be looking at what I was eating and usually say something like: "Now Steve, do you have any idea how many calories are in that meal?" She would then take out her iPhone and count the number of calories using an app on her phone. Kim could always make me laugh with her fat jokes such as "Now Steve, do you really need that chocolate? Let's look at how many calories are in that shall we". or "Steve, just think of how many hours you're going to have to spend on the treadmill to burn that meal off". Even though I was never proud of the way I looked, Kim always found a way to cheer me up and make me laugh.

I've always felt comfortable having these conversations around Kim. She knew exactly what I was going through and never made me feel down, even when things started to look grim, which in my case, was usually quite often.

In mid-2012 Kim was about to head overseas on an exchange program for Uni (she was studying to be a primary school teacher), and she was telling me that she badly wanted to get herself into shape before she went over there. I remember her telling me that she was about to start boot camp and asked me to come along with her. I reacted the same way I did when Hayley asked me to try it, I laughed and thought, no chance in hell.

Kim ended up doing a few sessions of boot camp and then, in the days following, she told me all about it and how much fun it was. She also told me about the pain that she was enduring afterwards. All I could think was thank God I never went through with it.

In September 2012, Kim was still in the U.S, and as I started losing more weight I began posting my progress shots on Facebook. After a couple of days there was a comment from Kim saying that I looked awesome. Now that was a great feeling, it gave me motivation to go on. As the months went on, Kim continued to share her support and kind words of inspiration which have, to this day, like many others, still kept me motivated to keep going on my weight loss journey.

Kim returned back to work in February 2013 after being gone for almost seven months. By that stage I had lost close to 30kgs and when Kim saw me for the first time since she returned, she looked at me and smiled with joy and said: "Steve, you look amazing".

I am very proud to have met all these inspirational people who all share a special part in my life.

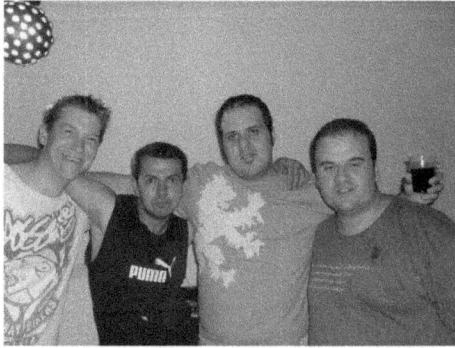

Jason Guthrie, Chris Lindsay, Anthony Epifanio and me
at a New Year's Eve event in 2009.

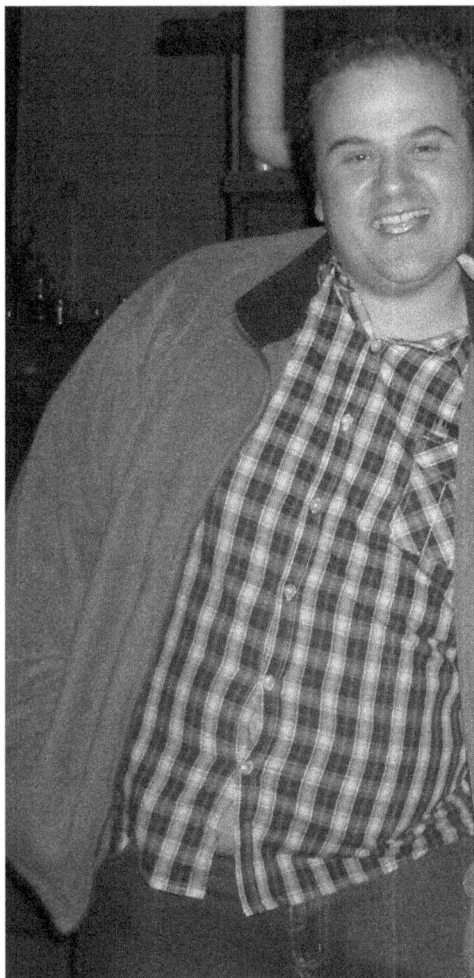

At my 30th birthday in April 2011. I weighed over 130kgs.
A pretty disturbing image, but a reflection of what my life once was.

Chapter 9

Village Cinemas and Payless Shoes

In November 2009 I was only working a casual job for a local service station and I was under a lot of financial strain. I needed a full-time job but no one seemed to be looking for full-time workers.

One day I was walking through a newly opened shopping centre in South Morang and I walked past a store that was advertising a casual sales position. I walked into the store, known as Payless Shoes, and spoke to the store manager regarding the position.

I filled out the application and afterward went home and hoped for the best. That same night, I decided to also look for work online in case there was anything full-time in another industry. As I searched through the Internet, I noticed that Village Cinemas were also hiring casuals. I tried my luck and applied for that job also, not really expecting to hear anything, as I had always loved the movies, but never managed to get a job with the company.

A couple of days later I got a phone call from the boss at Payless Shoes who called me in for an interview. I went down to the centre and met the manger in the food court for my interview. We were talking for what seemed like hours, perhaps the longest one on one interview I have ever had. The manager seemed pretty impressed with my interview and told me that if I was successful I would find out by the end of the week.

The following day, at home, I was going through my emails and noticed that I had only one email in my junk folder. It was just by chance that I checked my junk folder as it is usually full of spam. When I opened the folder I saw that Village Cinemas had responded to my application and I had been accepted for a group interview session to be held that same Saturday morning.

On Friday afternoon I received a phone call from the manager at Payless Shoes telling me that I was successful with my application and she offered me the job of a casual store assistant.

Even though I got the job with Payless Shoes I decided to go to the group interview for Village. I wasn't really concerned if I didn't get the job as I had already been successful with Payless. When I arrived, I remember being in a room with about fifteen or twenty other people. The group interview went for two hours and we were told that if we

49

were successful we would find out within the next few days.

I remember sitting in the food court at the centre, I must have had my phone on silent because the next thing I remember, I was looking down at my phone and noticed a missed call. I didn't recognise the number so I called it back. When I eventually got through, it was the manager from Village Cinemas telling me that I had also got the job as a casual assistant.

It was never my intention to work two jobs, but they both came at such an ideal time. By April 2010, I was made permanent part-time with Payless Shoes as an assistant store manager. I was averaging 30 hours per week with Payless and knowing that my hours were on a permanent basis, I was able to juggle both jobs without either of them interfering with the other. I started employment with Village Cinemas at a small site and I was only trained in the Gold Class area. In September 2010, I moved to a much busier site and got trained in all aspects of the business.

In January 2011, I became permanent part-time with Village, also averaging about 25–30 hours per week.

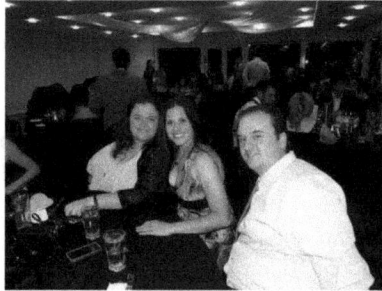

From left to right, Rebecca Andrews, Tina Gephart
and me at our staff party in March 2012.

Chapter 10

Back To Titanic

April 2012 not only was my 31st birthday, but it also marked the 100th anniversary of the *Titanic's* maiden voyage and its fateful sinking. To commemorate this, *Titanic* the movie was re-released in theatres in 3D. At Village, we were showing *Titanic* in Gold Class so I hired out the cinema for my party. When the film was released over 16 years ago, I saw it in excess of 20 times at the cinemas and to this day, it still remains my all-time favourite movie. I jumped at the chance to see it again in cinemas.

In theme of the commemoration, I decided for my birthday that year, to have a fancy dress party. Those invited, were required to dress in 1912 attire as if they were attending a first class dinner on board the ship in 1912. I had done my research and I wanted to make sure that I looked perfect and have the exact attire for the occasion.

I had started a diet and lost some weight and was hopeful that I would find something that was going to fit; the only thing was, I didn't have a clue where to get it from. I then heard an ad on the radio advertising the *Titanic* Theatre Restaurant which was located in Williamstown. I drove down there the next day to check it out and was surprised at what I found. The restaurant's interior was designed just like the *Titanic*. It wasn't an exact replica, but so much detail had gone into the design to make it look as it did back in 1912. At the top of the restaurant was the 'Captain's Quarters'. The owner of the restaurant lived upstairs which again was designed and built to look like the ship's captain's quarters in 1912.

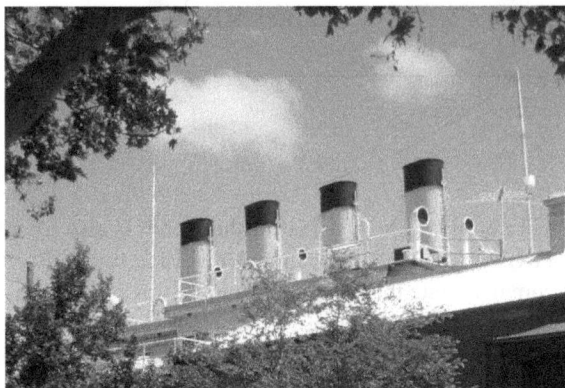

The "Captains Quarters" on top of the *Titanic* Theatre restaurant in Williamstown.

The restaurant caters for many occasions, is open for lunch and dinner and has a great theatre show. One Saturday night I went and had dinner at the restaurant with a group of friends and afterwards we went downstairs or 'Third Class' as it was known on the ship. While you are downstairs in 'Third Class' you stand on a wooden floor which has glass in the middle of it. At approximately 10:00pm the glass section of the floor fills with water and 'floods' and the floor pivots up and down as if actually sinking. You are given life jackets as part of the show as well.

I needed a tuxedo that I could wear for my party. The restaurant had almost every outfit you could think of for 1912. I tried on the tuxedo that the owner of the restaurant showed me and he told me that the sizes were smaller than normal. *Yes!* It just fitted, it was a little tight around the waist, but I could handle it. There were still a few weeks until the party so I was even more determined to lose some more weight to make this outfit fit.

I remained committed to my diet, I had a goal and I worked damn hard towards it. Fitting into that tux meant more to me than anything and that was my motivation. I wanted to look good for my birthday. After all, I didn't want to be upstaged by anyone else, and this was my night.

I made sure that I could get myself down to that size so that I could look good. By the time my birthday arrived on April 10th, 2012, I lost 12kgs and I was able to fit into that tuxedo perfectly.

I always hated photos because they made me look fat and I was never happy with my image. On that night I was much happier, I was actually smiling and, for once, I looked really good in a suit. Six weeks prior to my birthday was the staff party and everyone could see what a difference 12kgs made to my image. I hadn't reached my goal by any means, but I started to look and feel good for the first time in ages.

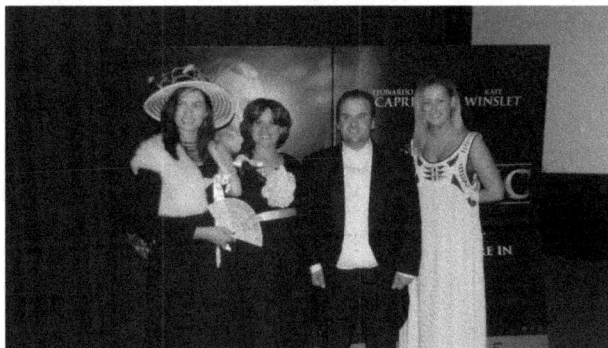

Hayley Griffiths, Tina Gephart, me and Lauren Whitty, on the night of my 31st birthday. The final result,12kgs lighter and all dressed up in 1912 attire for *Titanic* celebrations.

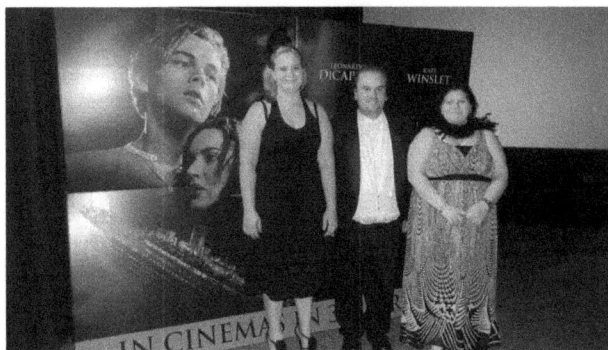

Sarah Bell, me and Loretta Bell at my *Titanic* celebrations, 12kgs lighter and starting to look in much better shape.

I had a lot of fun that night, but once the night was over I was once again left all alone. The hardest thing for me was that I had feelings for a colleague of mine, but I was too scared to act on those feelings.

I hadn't been with a woman for so long and I didn't know how to ask a girl out because I spent most of my life confused.

Rejection was my biggest fear. I could never handle being rejected. I was always afraid of asking a girl out in case she said no and I didn't know how I would react to it. I never ended up asking the girl out. I cared about her too much and didn't want to lose her as a friend. We were so close and I didn't want to jeopardise that by telling her how I felt, so I kept my feelings to myself. I don't regret not asking her out, but I constantly ask myself "What if?" What if I did ask her out? Who knows where my life would be at now?

Chapter 11

Late Night Snacks, Binging and the Final Straw

I spent most of my life growing up as a large kid and I always loved my food. I loved my job at Village, but it did have its downfalls. One of those was that at most times, my shifts were usually starting at around 6pm because I was working at Payless Shoes until 5 or 5:30pm. Usually, if I started a shift at 6pm it meant that I never had time for dinner as I was travelling from one job to the other.

Travelling between the two jobs and late nights meant that I had no time to prepare any of my meals so I was always going to Village without food. I would always wait for my break time and then head down to the food court and buy my dinner from there. I always used food as a form of comfort, not even thinking about what I was doing.

I think it was more psychological, my mind was always telling me to eat even when I wasn't hungry. Most nights, even after I had eaten a big meal at work, I would get home and eat again. It was always straight to the fridge to see what was in there, sometimes it was a block of chocolate or pizza. Other times I got lucky with the previous night's left overs. After eating all that, I would usually head straight off to bed bloated, letting all the food in my stomach stay there and store itself as fat.

Even as I lay there at night feeling sick, I still ignored the reality of who I was. I wasn't happy. I wasn't happy because I had nothing, no girlfriend, no money, and no confidence. After all these years I was still confused and I was trying to live a lie.

Whenever I lost weight, I always put it back on much faster and I put more of it on than what I originally lost to begin with. Whenever that happened, I would always try and cover it up by wearing clothing that was even bigger than I was to try and hide my true size. I avoided everything because I just did not have the help and support that I needed to help me through.

When attending functions, I always kept to myself because I never fitted in. Everyone at these parties either had a partner or was a lot thinner than I was. At times I thought of not going to many of these functions, but I was always invited by people who I was friends with, so out of respect I always went to them.

In July 2012, I was invited to attend Theresa's 30th birthday party.

Her theme was music and we all had to get dressed up as someone in the music industry. It was really hard for me to try and find an outfit that I would look good in and so I took the easy way out. I had a black shirt, jeans and some glasses; all I needed was a wig. In the end I went as Ozzy Osbourne, the only thing I could think of that could cover what I felt 'uncomfortable' showing.

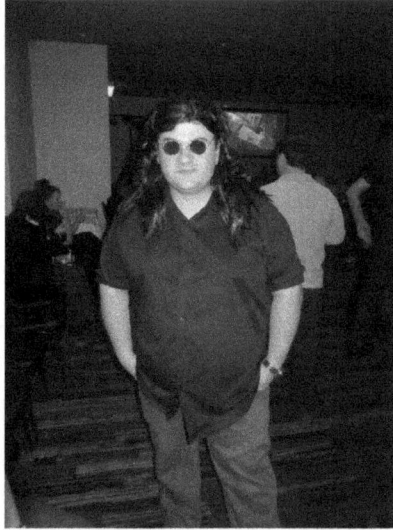

Taken at Theresa Lindsay's 30th birthday party in July 2012 dressed as Ozzy Osbourne. At the time of the party I had already put back on 10 of the 12kgs that I had lost for my birthday in April and I looked really unhealthy.

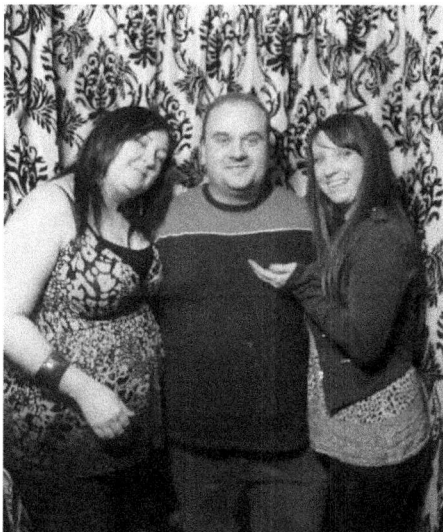

Joan Wallace, me and Theresa Lindsay. This photo was taken less than four weeks after Theresa's birthday and I had put on another 5kgs, taking me back over 130kgs. Out of all the photos throughout my life, I would have to say that this would be the most difficult one for me to look at.

Chapter 12

Catarina Fernandes

In February 2012, I had been working for Payless Shoes for just over two and a half years. A management opportunity arose at one of our smaller stores and my district manager put me up for the position. From February to the end of August that year I managed the store, but with the stress of the position and my personal life, I started putting more weight on.

I knew I had to do something, I was getting out of control, but I had no one around for support or motivation. I couldn't talk to my parents about it because I never had the help and support that I so desperately needed. I had no one that I could turn to for guidance.

After the store that I was managing closed down, I was given the opportunity to work at another store to relieve the assistant manager who had gone overseas for six weeks. On September 10th, 2012, I walked through the doors of Payless Shoes in Broadmeadows.

This is where it all happened, things changed, my life changed, I know that sounds kind of cliché but it's true. Looking back, this is where I made one of the best decisions to truly take control of my weight and my physical and mental health.

The manager of that store was the one who made that life-changing phone call to me. She asked for me personally as she had previously worked with me at another store that she managed, and she knew that I was capable of doing the job. Catarina Fernandes came into my life at just the right time.

I sat down and had a chat with Catarina (Cat) in her first ever exclusive one on one interview where I openly spoke to her for the first time about my personal struggles with weight loss. Also, Cat talks about how she helped me lose weight and why she enjoyed it so much.

Steve: Cat, first of all, how did you and I first meet (before Broadmeadows)?

Cat: We first met at the Northland store that I was managing at the time; you and I talked over the phone many times. When I first heard your voice I already pictured you to look a certain way, I guess we all do this. We normally picture someone to look a certain way before actually seeing them. Well one day you came to Northland with your mother and introduced yourself as being Steve from South Morang (Plenty Valley).

S: And how long ago was that?

C: We met about three years ago in 2010.

S: When you first saw how big I was, what was going through your mind?

C: Steve when I first saw you, like I said before, I pictured you to look a certain way, and when I saw you for the first time, that wasn't what I was expecting. I thought to myself, "geez, he's a big boy and I can't believe he's only 29 years old, he looks older, what the hell is he eating, maybe I can help him".

S: My weight and image has always been a struggle for me. Why do you think I have struggled so much to lose weight and keep it off?

C: You have struggled because all you did was eat crap, crap and more crap, you were binge eating. I think your personal life and everything that was happening around you affected your weight. So the only way to make you feel better about yourself was by eating crap every day.

S: You've always been someone who has taken health and fitness seriously. Why is it so important to you?

C: It's important to me because you are what you eat, and image is a big thing these days. Health is also important because if we don't have health we have nothing. I love educating people about health and fitness; it makes me feel whole knowing I can help someone achieve goals they never knew they could accomplish.

S: On September 10th, 2012, I came to your store to relieve your 2IC who was overseas at the time and it was there where my whole journey started. What can you tell everyone out there about that day when I first admitted to you that I had a problem and I needed your help?

C: The first thing I said was it's about f@#*@#% time, thank God you have realised this. I actually thought that you were only just saying that you wanted to lose weight and I didn't actually think you'd go ahead with it. I said to myself, "It's probably a waste of time, but I'm still going to try and help". You asked me to write you up a food plan and I did.

S: You inspired me to make this change in my lifestyle. How does it make you feel knowing that you inspired me to change my lifestyle?

C: It makes me feel great cause that's what I do. I always try and educate people that I care about, how to live a healthy lifestyle; I guess it also makes me feel special knowing that I was a part of your continuous success.

S: I remember you telling me that no matter what happens (in the event that you ever left the company) make sure I stick to the diet. What can you remember about that conversation?

C: I remember telling you that I really wanted you to succeed. So I made sure that you understood that I cared for you and wanted to help you even though I wasn't there. I also remember saying to you that I was going to bust your balls and that I would call you from my new job to check up on you. I knew then that from that moment, I had made an impact on you.

S: Looking back over my journey, did you honestly think I would listen to your advice and stick to it?

C: No! I thought to myself "this guy isn't going to stick to this food plan and exercise program, no way" I actually thought that you didn't care about how you looked; you were just comfortable being the way you were.

S: Talk me through that day at work where you made lunch and dinner for me. Why did you do it?

C: I made you lunch and dinner because I wanted to show you, 1– how food should look and teach you portion sizes, 2– that it is easy to cook homemade meals and 3– I'm a great cook, so I just wanted you to taste my food. I cared about you and I wanted to teach you how to change your eating habits.

S: Throughout this journey you have been, and continue to be, yet another inspiration in my life that has made me succeed. How do you think you have inspired me to get this far?

C: I have inspired you by telling you the truth that no one else had the heart to tell you. I remember you were in the back room at work eating lunch and we were having a conversation and I said to you "Steve, I can only do so much, you need to want to do this, and there is no point me talking about it and you do nothing about it. At the end of the day, you're the one looking the way you do, not me". I think from that day onwards you looked at life with different eyes.

S: In this book I talk about stress, self-esteem and lack of confidence as the main reasons why I put on weight. Do you think there is more to it than that?

C: Yes!!! I think your family and personal life played a great part in it, and the fact that you didn't have a partner at the time or couldn't take girls out on dates made it hard for you too because you had been rejected so many times before.

S: What can you say, in your own words, about the results you have seen through my journey?

C: I was blown away, I was shocked, but at the same time I was proud of you, you stuck to everything that I had taught you and you succeeded.

S: I've mentioned to you now that I am going to become a Personal Trainer. What do you think about that?

C: At first I thought "how typical" (laughs), but I kind of suspected that once you had seen the results for yourself you would want to educate others in the same way that I did.

S: Did you have any doubts that I would succeed?

C: Yes! Absolutely, I had many doubts. I thought it was just a phase you were going through because you were working with me and you just wanted to fit in and be accepted. At the time, I didn't think you had it in you though. You were full of shit!

S: Are you proud of me?

C: F@#%, Shit yeah, oh my god. I tell everyone about your transformation, and that I was happy to help.

S: Can you describe my success in 10 words?

C: Steve, I can't describe it in 10 words but I can describe it in one word: *dedication.*

S: What do you think of the new me now?

C: The new Steve is fantastic; he's confident, and full of self-esteem.

S: Cat, you are the reason I started this journey in the first place and I will always be grateful to you. How can I repay you?

C: Steve, I have told you this many times before, I only guided you to follow a new path. I have done nothing, remember, you're the one that has done this, the only way that you can repay me is by staying true to yourself.

S: Do you think that I will be a great role model and inspiration to others, and if so, how?

C: Yes! I think you will be an amazing role model for others because you have a story to tell. You've been through it and have done all the hard yards to get to where you are today.

S: Finally, as I reach the end of this chapter in my life, what final words would you like to say to me?

C: Thank you for allowing me to guide you to a whole new life; it was an honour and a pleasure.

S: Thanks Cat.

I was lying in bed one night going through Facebook and I saw a comment that my cousin had posted. It was about a friend of hers and she was talking about all this weight that she had lost. She had been on this product that I had never heard of before for a week and she had lost 5 kilos. I thought nothing of the post at first and then went straight to bed.

The next night I was, once again, lying in bed reading another post that my cousin had put on Facebook. Again to my surprise there was a mention of a friend who had lost weight on this product. This person had lost 8 kilos in 2 weeks, there was something going on, "what is this product?" I kept saying to myself. I wanted to know more about it, so I sent my cousin an email and asked her what all this fuss was about. She told me about this product that she had discovered and told me to come over and see her one Friday night after work where she would tell me more about it.

I was still living at home with my parents at the time, and it was hard to buy my own foods and not eat Mum's cooking. Dad always had this thing about us eating other foods when Mum had made a home cooked meal.

I had been doing so well with the diet and I didn't want to ruin what I had already achieved. I started doing my own shopping, buying my own ingredients and preparing my own meals. I continued tomaintain my diet and kept losing weight at a healthy rate while still eating minimal amounts of Mum's food at dinner time.

The following day, I moved out of Mum and Dad's house in Eden Park. I was surrounded by stress and constant arguing; this wasn't a healthy lifestyle for me. It also didn't do anything for my confidence or my self-esteem and it was a major factor in my constant fluctuation with my weight all my life.

I had no support at home. I knew that if I stayed, I would never achieve the results that I wanted and I would never stop feeling sorry for myself.

I moved away, only 30 minutes down the road from Eden Park back to our old house in Epping. I was away from all the stress and constant negativity in my life and I could start concentrating on getting my health and fitness in order and start living a healthier and happier lifestyle.

Chapter 13

September 2012

Catarina had resigned from Payless and I was now on my own. I remained at the store for a further 2 weeks until my business manager called to tell me that I would be returning back to my home store in Plenty Valley. By now, I had lost close to 8kgs in total, but personally I couldn't tell because I looked at myself every day and I still looked the same.

Nevertheless, I maintained my diet and kept my promise to Catarina, I continued to eat healthy and cut down on my portion sizes. I had moved out of home which meant that I could now prepare all my own meals which were much healthier. Keeping up with this new habit I started to see results, the weight kept dropping off and I was starting to look good and feel better about myself as well. I also started to get my confidence back.

It's no secret that I hated exercise, the best thing was that I continued to lose weight even without exercising or any form of fitness training. The loss was slow, but losing weight slowly was always better than losing it quickly as there was always the risk of putting the weight back on just as fast. Even when I was back at Plenty Valley, the temptation to eat junk food had suddenly disappeared.

I was determined to stick this one out. I set my mind towards something and I went for it, making sure that I didn't let anything, or anyone get in my way. The one thing that I was looking forward to in September was a family wedding. My mother's first cousin was getting married and their wedding was coming up. I loved weddings, but I certainly didn't love dressing up for them as nothing would fit. I never looked as good as my Dad or my brothers.

September 8th had arrived and my Mum's cousins were married. Catarina, picked out a shirt for me and I managed to scrub up ok, even though the shirt I was wearing was a size 6XL. The biggest shirt size I had ever worn. Even after losing about 8kgs I still couldn't manage to fit into anything smaller without feeling uncomfortable.

I remember sitting at the table that night, I sat directly opposite my parents so that I could hide away from Dad. The thing that is hard about weddings, especially European ones, is the amount of food that you eat. I had lost some weight, and I thought to myself, was I really going to deprive myself of food just because I was on a diet, especially at a wedding? No. So I didn't. I ate all the meals that were served that night and I did feel a little guilty afterwards. Even though I knew it was only for one night and tomorrow I would be straight on the diet again, it didn't help that sinking feeling knowing what I had just eaten.

That night, my Mum's cousins Chris Karakaltsas and Sue Christov had just flown back in from Las Vegas to attend the wedding. It had been years since I had last seen either of them and they both looked different compared to the last time we had all seen each other. I couldn't quite work out what it was at the time. It wasn't until Chris and Sue came to our table to say hello and that's when my mother and grandmother both noticed that Sue had lost weight.

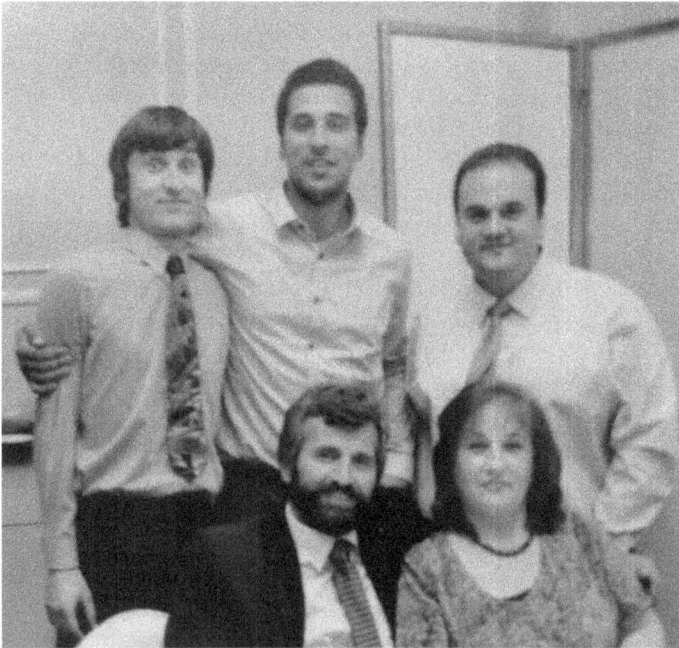

Paul, Christopher, me, Dad and Mum at a Wedding in September 2012.

We had almost hit the end of September and I was still losing weight at a comfortable rate. At work things also started to change, my closest friends and colleagues had started to notice the changes in me and started to compliment me for the way I looked.

It was the best feeling I had had in a very long time. The cravings had also gone. I no longer craved fast foods or any junk food for that matter. I cut out soft drinks and sweets completely and also reduced my bread intake, which was hard.

Carbohydrates are the biggest killer in all diets, and for me, being European, I loved bread, but like everything else I cut it out. By now I had been on the diet for close to 4 ½ weeks and I knew what portions I was meant to be having for my meals.

This was the hardest thing I had to adapt to, as my stomach had now started to shrink. If I ate too much, I started to feel sick, unlike before when my body just wanted more.

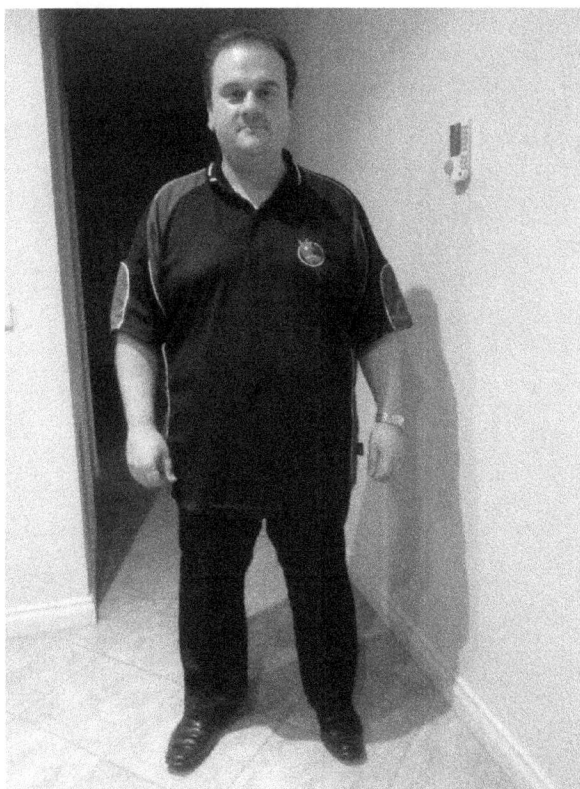

The final 'before' shot, taken at the end of September just before I started on the Herbal products and Personal Training. I was really nervous and didn't know what to expect of this product that I had heard so much about.

Chapter 14

Sue Christov and Chris Karakaltsas

The night had arrived for my meeting with my cousin. Sue is married to my mother's first cousin, Chris Karakaltsas and the two of them live in Mill Park. It was 9:30pm on a Friday night and I had just finished my shift at work and I headed over to Sue's house.

When I arrived, Sue spent hours talking to me about the Herbal products. I had never heard about the product and only knew of it through the posts on Facebook. Sue briefly went through the product and its history, which spans back more than 30 years. She was very passionate about the product which has helped her achieve amazing success.

Sue and Chris started on the program back in June 2012, when it was introduced to them by former Carlton AFL Footballer, Anthony Koutoufides, who started taking the product 1 year before that.

Since starting the program in June 2012, Sue had lost 15kgs and Chris had lost 12 by September, after only being on the program for three and a half months. Sue started telling me about how amazing she looked and how the product made her feel fantastic and gave her so much energy. I guess we only ever hear about these success stories from celebrities and people that have large amounts of cash, who can afford surgery or personal training.

Not Sue however, she showed me some photos of her and Chris before they started this program and I can tell you the results speak for themselves when you compare the differences. I couldn't believe what I was seeing and it was all right in front of my eyes. It truly was amazing, I hadn't known Sue for very long at this stage, and I was very sceptical about trying this product that I barely knew anything about.

Sue explained the product to me and she was clearly living proof that the product was working, but what about side effects, long term health problems and all that? I kept asking myself these questions out of concern that it might be too good to be true.

After seeing the results on Chris and Sue I was satisfied that the product was safe to use. They had both been on it for over six months and neither of them had had any health related issues whilst using the product. That's all that I needed to know at that stage. I was desperate and I would try anything to lose weight and clearly, judging from Sue and Chris's results, it was working.

The most difficult thing for me that night was opening up to Sue about my struggles over the years and not just about weight loss. Although I hadn't known Sue very long, she was family and probably, at that point, the only person who was family that I could really talk to. I had never been able to talk to my immediate family about the problems I had been through; probably because my family may have been the cause of my struggles.

The hardest thing for Sue that night was digesting the information that I had just told her. That's when she made the decision that she was going to help and support me through this part of my life. Having already started my own diet, I was already going onto this program with a head start. I had already lost close to 10kgs and it was time for Sue to introduce me to the Herbal products and get me started.

I had used a couple of different scales to measure my weight loss. The results fluctuated from time to time, depending on what scales I was using. I was nervous as hell, but at the same time, I was really excited and anxious to start this product and start seeing the results. Before the night ended, Sue put me on the advanced program and took my weight and measurements.

I had only heard about this product through Sue, not in the media, not in books or anything, even though it had been around for over 30 years. I decided to get the inside story on Sue. I wanted to know about her success and more about this amazing product that was such a success to everyone using it.

In an emotional interview, Sue and I chat in the comfort of her home about her life before the Herbal products, meeting Chris and getting married. Sue opens up to me about the difficult struggles she faced on her journey. She also explains how this product has now changed not only hers and my life, but most importantly, the lives of others.

Steve: Sue, you look amazing and congratulations on your great success. How does it feel, looking back on all your old photos and clothing, knowing how much weight you have lost and what you have achieved?

Sue: Thank you Steve, wow, Oh My God, yep I am very proud of myself. When I look at all the old photos I think oh my God how did I let myself get to that point? But I did, I got complacent and comfortable in my skin at the time. But now looking back at it all, I think "what a journey, what an achievement". Everyone around me is proud, my friends, my family, oh and most importantly my husband (Chris). He takes photos of me and he wants me to put them all over Facebook. So there you go.

S: So Sue, I guess the most important question to ask is; how did you find out about this product?

Sue: Back in February 2012, I was at Anthony and Suzie (Koutoufides') house with my hairdresser and Anthony had just vaguely approached me and mentioned these Herbal products and that my hairdresser and I should get onto it. We both just totally avoided him and didn't really take much notice. It was then about six months later in June, when Peter (Damevski) and Anthony had been talking. Peter had started to get involved with the Herbal products and he was the one that actually approached me, and Steve. At that point he scared me. He scared me by telling me that we (Chris and I) were overweight and we were candidates for heart attacks and diabetes and things like that and that scared us a lot. So that's what prompted me to start. Then Anthony got on board and had a bit of a chat to us, he went over the program with me and that's how we found out about the Herbal products; well the Herbal products found us actually.

S: Sue, were you happy with your life before starting the Herbal products?

Sue: Steve, honestly, I thought I was. I threw out all of my skinny clothes and I thought, being so big, that the journey ahead for me to start dieting and exercising was going to be hard. It was going to be hard because it was such a big challenge and I didn't really think of it. No actually, to tell you the truth, I didn't even want to do it. I was quite happy, everyone in my family is big, my sister is big my mother was a bit largish and I thought to myself, well this is my life. I've found the love of my life and we are both going to grow old and fat together and we were happy with that. I never even thought to try and lose weight because the journey was going to be so hard, but with Herbal products, I found it extremely easy and I thank one man for that and that's Mr. Koutoufides.

S: What made you want to do something about your weight and image?

Sue: I guess, Steve, when it was presented to me all the diseases that I could get, heart attacks, diabetes and high cholesterol, it was an eye opener. I'm not one to take medication and I didn't want to live the rest of my life taking medication and being drugged up. Another thing Steve, to tell you the truth, the hardest thing about it all, and I don't talk about this very much, but, it was also the issue of buying clothes. It was very hard to buy clothes because I would see a beautiful looking dress on a mannequin and it would look immaculate, then I would walk into the shop and I could never find my size. If I did end up finding my size, it never looked the same and I always tried to cover my weight or somehow make it work so that I looked ok. The reality was that they were never my style of dresses, but I adapted to it. So I guess I can say that it was my clothing and my health that made me do this.

S: Your husband (Chris) is also on the program, did he want to try this product to lose weight as well or did he just do it to support you because you were doing it?

Sue: No, he wanted to do it together so that we could support each other. He was all for it, he was actually the one that convinced me to go on the product and pushed me onto it. So we both started doing it together.

S: Can you tell us what you weighed before starting the program?

Sue: *(Laughs)* Yep, I was 88.5kgs and that was in June 2012, and now in 2013 I'm at 65, so a total loss of 23.5kgs in approximately 10 months.

S: Did you always struggle with your weight and image in the past?

Sue: Um, yes and no Steve. This is kind of hard to explain, growing up, I was always a skinny little thing. If I put on a bit of weight I wasn't happy about it so I would quickly go on a diet or start exercising. I only did that if I put on 6–10kgs though, but this time, I let my weight go too far for me to do anything about it. Previously, I could say that I did put on weight, but it wasn't excessive, and mind you I wasn't happy with even putting on a little bit of weight so I would fix it. So I can say that I wasn't always overweight.

S: Did you try any other diets before Herbal products?

Sue: This time around (before starting on the Herbal products) No! Previously, yes. I tried everything, the healthy eating, and cutting down on foods, but I always felt lethargic and I got really tired of it. I had been exercising and going to the gym and all that stuff and I was really good too, I maintained it. However, I wasn't getting the proper nutrients from food. I would lose the weight and then I would get tired and I would be hungry again. I would then go back to eating and start putting the weight back on and the worst part, this time I put it on 3 times as much.

S: How has the product changed your life (other than the obvious)?

Sue: Oh My God *(laughing)*, where do I start Steve? Well first of all the inner world. I'll talk about the inner self, I feel so much healthier, and the energy (I'm 49 this year) and for my age, the energy levels are just *wow*, gone through the roof. I'm very energetic, always on the go, on the inside I feel fantastic, and from the outside...

S: You look great...

Sue: Thank you. Yeah I think I look good *(laughs)*. The best thing about all this is the fact that I'm 49 and my metabolic age is 34 at the moment which is marvellous considering when I started, it was 64. I not only look good, but I also feel good, I can finally fit into clothes that I want to wear, I have no problems going up and down stairs anymore, and I don't get out of breath. Steve, the best thing of it all is that I have started to exercise and I am doing fit clubs and keeping up with all the advanced people.

Since losing the weight I am able to exercise, whereas prior, when

I was carrying all the weight I didn't want to exercise because I couldn't cope. I was huffing and puffing, I couldn't run or even jog whilst carrying 88kgs. Being so big, that's what deterred me from losing weight previously, but now, I feel fantastic, I feel like a spring chicken.

S: You mentioned you were doing fit clubs, can you tell us what Fit Club is all about?

Sue: Anthony (Kouta) takes Fit Club. There is a group of us and we are all at different fitness levels, so we all do it at our own pace. It consists of running, circuit exercising, and it's a lot of fun, but what I must say is that it is not boot camp, he doesn't yell or scream at us. It's a social gathering. We've all made a lot of friends and it's like a little connection that we all have, everyone supports each other.

S: Sue, this is a tough one, but were you hesitant to try the product?

Sue: *(Pause)* you're right, that is a tough one Steve, if I had to make the decision on my own I would say yes.

No, because my husband pushed me, actually not pushed me as such, he was very supportive of it, he wanted to do it, so we did it together. If I was on my own Steve, yeah I probably would have been hesitant because I would have been alone. Peter and Anthony had shown me other people's results, but I was still hesitant. Chris was the main motivator in my life at the time and we've been doing it together and succeeding.

S: So Sue, we now all know about you and your history with your weight and these Herbal products. We are now going to talk about me and my success on the product because there are people out there who want to know how I got to where I am today.

Sue: Sure, go right ahead.

S: You signed me up on the program back in September 2012. Why do you think I chose to come to you instead of someone else for help?

Sue: Well because I'm your gorgeous hot cousin *(laughing)*. I think you came to me because you had seen Chris and me at a family wedding after we returned from our trip to Vegas. I think that's what did it for you. I remember you initially contacting me through Facebook and telling me that I looked amazing, what am I on, I want this stuff.

I made an appointment with you and we took it from there. I think seeing the results on Chris and me and being related made you feel more comfortable with me, being able to talk to me and, of course, me being a female and the lovely person that I am *(laughing)*.

S: This is going to take you back a little. What can you tell every-body out there about our first meeting together?

Sue: I remember you walking through my front door, and I saw a very enthusiastic, scared, not to mention excited young man walk before me, a very overweight young man. However, it was the enthusiasm in you that really stood out, especially in your eyes; it was also your determination. We sat down and had quite a long talk, I explained the product to you, how it all worked in detail and I encouraged you to try it. I told you that I was going to be there to support you, and that no matter what, you could always call me at any time, day or night which of course you have. I saw the want in your face, in your eyes, you wanted to do this, and at the same time I could see you were hesitant and the whole "am I doing the right thing, what is this stuff", I think you seeing my results was what you needed to get started.

S: Sue, I came to you weighing over 120kgs (Oh My God!). What was going through your mind after my first consultation and the results were, let's just say not so good?

Sue: Well when I got you on the scales Steve it wasn't so much the weight, even though it was an obvious thing that the weight was there. However, what scared me the most Steve, and I'll be very hon-est with you, was the visceral fat which, for everyone out there, is the fat around your heart. The visceral fat causes heart attacks, blocked arteries and all sorts of things. For someone of your age to have such a high reading of 22, at the time was scary. I must mention though, that you have now brought this down, and I am so proud of you. With the visceral fat, anything over 13 is alarming; everything else really didn't matter to me. Actually, I should mention the body fat, that did matter to me, but it was more the visceral fat which was the most important. It was then when I realised that we really need to work hard here and we needed to do it together. I have to hand it to you though Steve, you did embrace it, you handled the readings really well, even though it wasn't good and we realised that we have a bit of work ahead of us. I remember explaining to you that you had to be patient because this wasn't going to happen overnight, it wasn't even going to happen in a month and you understood that which was really good. All I want to say to you Steve, is I am so proud of what you have done. Deep down, I knew you could do it because I saw the determination in your eyes and I heard it in your voice and I knew that you were going to do this. Most of all, it's what happened when you walked out of my house with the pack I had given you, it was the days that followed. You were calling me and texting me, I knew you had started the product and you were concerned because you wanted to make sure you were doing it correctly and that's why you were calling me. At that point I thought to myself, shit, this guy is going to do it and that's what made me more determined to be there for you. I know that along this journey Steve, I've been hard on you, telling you that you can't cheat; you can't do this and that, but at the end of the day, you're the one that needed to achieve this. I'm sure there were times when you probably hated me but, really, I don't think I was that harsh.

S: I have always struggled with my weight and image, and it's not something that I have been proud of. I've tried diets in the past but I've never stuck to them. Tell me how you think you made me stick to this product and the diet.

Sue: Simple. I was always on your back; encouraging you, motivating you, being your inspiration, by telling you that if I could do it, then you could do it. I think just being there for you and listening to you as well helped you when you needed me. You never ignored my phone calls; you never hung up on me and stuff like that. Being there and guiding you through the whole thing and encouraging you, well I think I encouraged you…

S: Definitely!

Sue: I kept saying to you, Steve don't give up, never ever give up. My advice to you is, whatever you do in life, don't give up. There might be times when it seems like you're going downhill, but never give up because there is always an upside to a downside.

S: You have regular follow-ups with all your clients who are on Herbal products. How often would you say you followed up on my progress?

Sue: *(Laughing).*

S: What's so funny?

Sue: Steve, I never had to follow up, you always followed up with me. *(laughing)...(still laughing)*

S: Sue, just say what you're going to say.

Sue: Like I said, I didn't really follow up with you because you stayed in touch with me a few times a day *(laughing again)*.

In all honesty, you were probably one of my easiest clients who I didn't have to follow up with *(laughing)*. Can we share your text messages with the public Steve?

S: Um no! Enough said let's move on. So after my first follow up consultation with you, can you tell everyone out there what results I had achieved and how you felt?

Sue: You had lost 6.1kgs, in exactly 4 weeks. The main thing that I felt (apart from being happy), was when I saw the look on your face. 6kgs in a month, your reaction was "Oh My God", I can't believe I have done this in such a short period of time. I knew that you could do it, because I know what the product does and how it works. I thought with all those phone calls and texts, something good had to have come out of that. I've been saying this to you throughout our whole conversation, but I am really proud of you Steve, you have done extremely well. I know you've struggled, and through those struggles, you know what, something good has come out of it now. It's made you a better and stronger person, a more confident person most of all. Oh My God, it just made me feel that, my work here is done. That's what it's all about, helping one person at a time and I didn't just help any person, I helped a cousin, family.

S: I've been on the product now for a while. What has it been like to watch me undergo a complete, major weight loss transformation right before your eyes?

Sue: It gives me pride, actually Steve; you are an inspiration to me when I see you do what you have done. I am really happy; no I'm extremely happy and very proud of you, a very big *proud*! At the same time I am happy for you because of how you feel, I can hear it, I can see it and you know you have done this. It's about your will power Steve, will power, it wasn't me or anyone else who did this, it was you. We've all been here to support and guide you, but you have done it all, so you need to say a *big* thank you to yourself and give yourself a big pat on your back. We (Chris, myself and Kouta), have been here to supply you with the tools, they are all there for you, but you're the one that has taken it all on board and done it. As much as I am proud of you Steve, you need to be proud of yourself as well.

S: The Herbal products have helped me achieve massive success and in such a short period of time. What advice can you give to other overweight people out there who are embarrassed with their image, sceptical about diets, and most importantly scared to make that first move?

Sue: Um, don't be scared. The Herbal products are simple, it's easy, and you can lose weight without exercising which I think is what puts a lot of people off. It is hard and you know that yourself, Steve, being a large person, that going straight into exercise is difficult after not doing it for so long. What I suggest is, don't be scared, others can look at the results that you have achieved and they can get themselves straight onto this product. They can lose the weight and get all their energy back because they are no longer carrying all that excess weight and they will be able to start exercising to be fit and healthy. The products are designed to lose weight without exercising and that's the way that I did it. You did it too; you lost a certain amount of weight at the start without exercising. You only just started doing intense training from November 2012 after being on the product for 6 weeks and you had already lost some weight. Exercising and healthy eating, as we all know is the best combination that you can get, so take the plunge, don't be scared and all they need to do is look at you if they have any doubts that this product works. Steve you, together with myself, my husband Chris, Kouta and 65 million people around the world, are all the product of the product. The results speak for themselves.

S: I know you have already answered this many times, but it's always good to hear it more than once. Are you proud of my success as well as your own?

Sue: Yes! Of course I am so proud of your success in a huge way. Remember you have done all this on your own Steve; we have been here to guide you and, support you, like I have already said, but you have done it on your own. I am very proud of you, Chris is proud of you; we all are because Steve, you are going to be an inspiration to others out there. In regards to my success, yeah, I'm happy, extremely happy, but at the end of the day I'm happier with your success Steve, because we've all achieved it together, but it is your success. You had a lot more weight to lose than I did, and that in itself is a lot harder. You have done that hard yakka let's just say, all the hard work, but in the end, you did, you're still doing it. It's fantastic no one could ever achieve this result and you have got all the people that love you and support you helping you do this. It's all because you want to do it Steve, nothing else. Be proud of yourself because as your family, Chris and I are both very proud of you. We are proud to be a part of your success and this whole transformation that we contributed to in a small way and that's what makes me happy.

S: Finally Sue, I saw you as my inspiration to lose weight and have a healthier lifestyle. How do you think I can inspire other people?

Sue: Oh My God are you serious kid? If you can't inspire other people out there then there is seriously something wrong. You have the personality, there is an aura about you that you will inspire other people, your results alone will inspire other people. This story of yours will inspire other people. What you have gone through and sharing it with the outside world will inspire others. Steve, there are people out there that are going through exactly what we have gone through. We have struggled with our weight, the negativity in our lives, as well as people putting us down. You have overcome all that, you're looking fantastic and that has to be all the inspiration that people need. You are going to inspire many people out there in a huge way and you will be changing people's lives and that's what makes me very proud of you. Steve, to you I say, good luck with the rest of your journey, you have done extremely well, and I know that the rest of your journey, not to mention the results, are going to be huge for you. Congratulations mate and we love you.

S: Thank you.

Chapter 15

The Herbal Products

By now, health and fitness started to play a key role in my life. I was surrounded by so many inspirational people and everyone was telling me that I started to look good. Even though I had started to lose weight I was still struggling with my personal issues. I had hoped that losing weight would have fixed the issues or at least make them easier; it didn't.

October 14th, 2012, just over two weeks had passed since I signed up on the program. I was still hesitant, I hadn't started the program yet, but I continued with my own diet and still watched what I was eating. I hadn't lost much more weight, but in saying that, I didn't put any weight on either which was a positive. At that stage, I had lost 11kgs in just over 6 weeks.

Three days later on October 17th, I started taking the Herbal Products. I remember talking with Anthony (Kouta) on Facebook and he was asking me how I was going on the product. I had only been on the product for one day and started to feel better already. As time went on I started getting used to the product, my cravings had stopped, I had much more energy and I was able to do things more easily without having trouble breathing.

By October 22nd, one week into the program, I had lost 2kgs on the Herbal products alone, bringing my total weight loss to 13kgs since starting the diet in September. I now started to feel good about myself and for the first time in many years my confidence and self-esteem also improved. I also started to look better at this point. I could finally start to see the results from the product and I started to get stricter with my eating and making more changes in my lifestyle.

By October 27th 2012, I had now lost 10kgs on the program and just over 20kgs in total. By now it was clear that the product was working and I could see some pretty impressive results and I was very happy.

I had started losing weight at a much slower rate at one point and I was getting angry and frustrated. I started thinking that maybe I was doing something wrong or not eating the right foods. I was constantly texting and calling Suzi and asked her if this was normal.

Suzi went through and explained to me that the body is going through massive changes and therefore it is adapting to those new changes, and as a result, the weight started to slow down, but I wasn't doing anything wrong.

We hit the end of October and I had been on the program close to three weeks. I continued to lose weight at a slow rate, but I was losing it all the same. It was my first week back at my original store in South Morang (Plenty Valley) after returning from my relief position at Broadmeadows with Catarina. At this stage, I had lost 12kgs on these Herbal products and almost 25kgs in total. The results were finally starting to show on my clothes at work, all my shirts started to feel loose and started to really look big on me.

I normally wore my pants on my hips and, being so big, I was never able to wear a belt as it constantly rubbed against the lower part of my stomach, but because my body was so big I never needed one. That was no longer a problem; I now started wearing my pants above my hips and up to my stomach which was something I had never done before. Even wearing my pants this high they were still loose. For the first time in many years, I had to finally start wearing a belt to keep my pants up, something I thought I would never be able to do again.

Saturday November 3rd, it was my first weekend back at my store and I was on my lunch break and I was walking through that food court where I would normally find it hard to fight the temptation to eat at a fast food outlet. Not anymore, I hadn't touched any sweets, junk food, soft drinks and I had substantially reduced my carbohydrate intake. I was controlling my cravings by drinking water and eating fruit. I was having small snacks during the day to avoid getting hungry and eating full meals.

On Monday November 5th, 2012 I had my first consultation for the Herbal products where we officially measured my results and progress. At one of these consultations, your coach, (in my case it was my cousin Suzi), does a monthly assessment on you where they measure your progress in specific detail. They measure things like your body fat, body water percentage, and muscle mass, BMR (Body Mass Range) which is similar to a daily calorie intake. They also measure your metabolic age.

Your metabolic age is the age at which your body is at, for example, in reality you could be 19 years old, but on the inside your body is functioning at a different age, normally much older if you are severely overweight like I was. They also measure your bone mass and visceral fat, which is the body fat that exists in the abdomen and surrounds the internal organs. The chart and information below breaks down, in detail, the results of my consultation whilst on the Herbal products:

Body Fat Range	% Body Water Range	Muscle Mass	Physique Rating	BMR	Basic Metabolic Age	Bone Mass	Visceral Fat
39	47.4	69.4	3	3501	46	3.6	22

Visceral Fat Range:

1–4   **Excellent**
5–8   **Healthy**
9–12   **Bad**
Over 13 **Alarming**

Metabolic Age:

The Metabolic Age rating indicates what age level your body is currently rated at:

Muscle Index and Physique Ratings:

Obese, Untrained	Normal	Exellent
1. Hidden Obese	4. Under Exercised	7. Thin
2. Obese	5. Standard	8. Thin and Muscular
3. Solidly-built	6. Standard Muscular	9. Very Muscular

The results show:
My Visceral Fat was **22** = **ALARMING**
My Metabolic Age = **46** (I'm only 32)
My Physique Rating = **3** which is **Solidly-built**

Age	Excellent	Healthy	Medium	Obese
20–24	10.8	14.9	19.0	**>23.3**
25–29	12.8	16.5	20.3	**>24.3**
30–34	14.5	18.0	21.5	**25.2**

Looking at this table you can compare my results below and you will see just how dangerously close I came to some very serious health issues:

My age is **32** and I have a Body Fat Range of **39** which = **OBESE** as it's over 25.2.

I headed into November with a better outlook on life, a new attitude and feeling great. By now I had learnt all about portion control, cravings and what foods I could and couldn't eat it. It had only been just over a month, but the results of this product were amazing and it was clearly starting to show.

Chapter 16

George Symeou and Personal Training

My biggest success through my weight loss hasn't only been about the Herbal products, although it was the key to most of my success it wasn't the only thing. The other important factor that contributed to my success was intense fitness training, exercise and a major change in my everyday lifestyle.

Overcoming my biggest demons and fears was never easy and probably one of the hardest things I ever had to do. I hated exercise and any form of physical activity; the thought of it made me cringe. Having already kick started my own health and fitness by dieting and using the Herbal products, I was on the road to good health. It was a Saturday afternoon and I was working with our casual at the time Nick Symeou, who was just 18.

I had heard about Nick and spoken to him many times previously over the phone, but this was the first time we had actually met face to face. Nick and I started talking and getting to know each other. He told me that he was studying graphic design at University, something he had a passion for. We then got into discussion about healthy eating and I started talking to Nick about all the weight I had been losing and how I was doing it.

He then asked me if I was seeing a personal trainer to which I replied no. The first thing I could think of was that time ten years ago when I was training with Josh and suddenly, all the memories and emotions came flooding back. Nick then explained to me that he had a twin brother George who, at 18, was already a fully qualified Personal Trainer.

A Personal Trainer at 18, I thought to myself, how is that possible? Nick explained to me that George had just got his qualification and was running his own gym from home and was always looking for new clients to take on.

I thought back to the time with Josh and it made me realise that I lost over 20kgs and I reached my target weight of 75–80kgs, surely I could do it again. I told Nick that I was interested and he gave me his brother's number. I called him up and organised a time for us both to meet face to face and discuss my fitness training. The following day, Sunday, George came down to my work and introduced himself as Nick's brother. We went out for a chat during my lunch break and I explained to George what I had already achieved on my own and the product that I was on. George went through his routines with me, how he works, his programs and the techniques of how he trains his clients to help them achieve their results.

I was so intrigued and amazed at his story and what he had achieved at such a young age. By the end of lunch I had signed up to do personal training with someone I had only just met, someone, who after 20 minutes, managed to convince me that they were going to give me results. George made a great first impression and I was drawn to his knowledge.

On Monday November 12th, 2012 I started my first personal training session. As it was my first session, George needed to know where I was at physically; he needed to do what we call 'Girth Measurements'. Girth Measurements are your progress results as you do personal training and George took my girth measurements every six weeks.

The following table shows exactly what my measurements were on my very first day of personal training. The table is substantially different to the Herbal products table. The Herbal products measure your progress from the inside as well as your weight, but the Girth Measurements measure your physical results on the outside.

Waist	Hips	Chest	Arms	Thighs	Calves
131cm	121cm	124.5cm	40cm	68cm	49cm

After my first session, I walked out of the gym feeling good and glad that I had taken that first initial step of my training. My first session mainly consisted of intense cardio, as this was going to speed up my weight loss.

There was a lot of hard work ahead of me. George and I agreed that for optimal results, ideally I should try and look at training three to four times a week in order to help speed up my metabolism and start getting my body back into shape. From then on, George and I trained four times a week, a consistency I maintained without fail. I never missed a session and if I did, it was either because I was sick or because of an extreme emergency situation.

I continued training and man was it tough, my body wasn't used to this kind of exercise after being absent from it for so long. There were many times when I just simply felt like giving up and just quitting. George remained strong and determined to get me through it. He kept pushing me to the max, making sure that I achieved what I so badly wanted. Intense cardio led to weight training which increased my body mass as I was gaining muscle.

Over the Christmas and New Year period, George took a week of holidays and made it very clear to me to make sure I maintained my exercises. He wrote me up a week's worth of exercises to do whilst he was away, including stretches.

This was perhaps the hardest part of the weight loss, not having George around to train me, and I knew that I was going to pig out over Christmas and suddenly I started to feel sick. I started to worry about what would happen if I got into that habit of bad eating again.

So Christmas and New Year came and George had returned from his holidays. Things were starting to get back to normal and I was starting to eat properly again.

I was so curious to know how bad I had done over the holidays because I knew I had eaten quite a bit. I jumped on the scales and found that over three weeks, where I let myself go a little bit, I had only managed to put on 1kg.

At first I thought there must be something wrong with the scales so I weighed myself again, nope, it was only a 1kg gain. I texted Suzi and told her straight away, I was so proud and happy at the same time. I had finally trained my body to consume food in moderation. Suzi too had told me that she put 2kgs on over Christmas and New Year, but she, like me, didn't let it get to her and we were more determined to lose it again so we started right back on being strict.

In January 2013, George was running outdoor classes for a week whilst his boss was on holidays. I mainly worked in the afternoons so I generally had the mornings free up until 11am. I always managed to fit in training before work. George was tied up with the outdoor training and it was hard to fit in my regular training sessions.

The only way George and I could find time to fit in my training was if I attended his outdoor sessions. It was still going to be one on one, but instead of it being indoors, we trained outside at a park. I didn't know what to expect from the class, but George set it up so that it was like a mini circuit which involved running with witches hats and hurdles. It also involved a bit of boxing as well as exercising using the medicine ball, doing the usual squats, lunges, push ups, sit ups, leg raises and bicycle kicks. It was kind of like a mini boot camp only without the yelling and no one else around. For the whole week I had two sessions outdoors and I have to admit, for something that I had never done before, other than P.E class at school, it really was interesting and a whole lot of fun.

At 18 years of age, George had already established himself as a personal trainer. Now, at 19, his business is growing rapidly. In the short time that I have known him, George has managed to give me a completely different outlook on health and fitness.

I sat down with George in his very first interview to find out more about his background, and how his hard work and dedication has helped change my lifestyle and inspired me to also start a career in fitness as a personal trainer.

Steve: George, the first question I want to ask you is what made you want to become a Personal Trainer?

George: Well when I was younger, I was a big kid about 60–70kgs at the age of 13. I used to get picked on at school and I had a lot of medical problems. One of those was high blood pressure and that's hereditary in my family; I didn't want to get to that as my family was unhealthy and unfit. The other thing is that I didn't want to get picked on so my twin brother and I went to school together. He used to get picked on more than I did and I couldn't take that. So I guess being fit, changed all that, I started getting bigger, more muscles and stuff like that. I started getting more confident and I started hitting it hard at the gym. I actually wanted to start helping people that were in my situation. It's something that I really enjoy doing, helping people get to their goals and everything that they want to achieve. I just started doing research and everything took off from there.

S: You mentioned you had a twin brother Nick, who I used to work with. Is he a trainer too?

G: No he is not a trainer; he and I are completely different.

S: Are you identical?

G: No we are not identical, but surprisingly we do look alike. We are what you call fraternal twins, meaning that we were both in different sacs when we were born, I came out first and then he came out second.

S: At the age of 18, most of us are busy looking at University options and what road we are going to take with our career. For you, at 18, you were already a fully qualified personal trainer. At what age did you know that you wanted to be a personal trainer?

G: At the age of 13 I purchased and owned my first set of dumbbells. That's when I started getting into the fitness. When I was about 15 I went overseas and I put on a shit load of weight, about 15kgs in total. When I came back I realised, WOW, time to get back into fitness so pretty much from the age of about 15 or 16 I knew that I wanted to be a trainer.

S: So you graduated from AIF (Australian Institute of Fitness), which is the school that Michelle Bridges from *The Biggest Loser* graduated from. What can you tell us about your time there?

G: It's probably the best thing that I have ever done. I knew what I wanted to do from Year 12, so I enrolled into the course, not really knowing what I was up for. It was in the city in Russell St and I attended the course twice a week. I did know some things, but they taught me a lot of new things and it made me more confident. I've met a lot of new people and made some amazing friends, it was a shame that I didn't meet Michelle, but I guess you can't have everything.

S: Ok, George so now we are going back to the time when you and I first met. In my story, I talk about the first time that I met you. What can you tell everyone about the first time you and I met?

G: Oh now that does take me back. I remember walking down to your work and meeting up with you, you seemed very keen to train. I didn't really know, at that time, if you were serious or not, or for that matter whether you actually took me seriously because I was only 18. I was keen and I remember you telling me that you had done personal training in the past, so it wasn't like we were going through the complete basics all over again. I didn't know what I could do or what you could do on a fitness level, so we arranged your first session and you came. I remember when I saw you, to me you looked, not upset, but not very happy either, you looked nervous and you didn't know what to expect. So I went through my usual consultations with you, I got to know what your goals were and what you wanted to achieve. I took your measurements and then we kicked off our first session. You seemed nervous, but the most important thing is, that you got through it and you did well. After the session, you and I had a chat and it was at that point when you let it all out. You talked to me about your self-consciousness, your self-esteem and how you let yourself go. From that point Steve, I clicked, I was like "nope, I'm going to help this guy".

S: When I first met you George back in November 2012, I told you what my goal was and what I wanted to achieve through weight loss and personal training. What was your reaction when you discovered just how much I weighed and the amount of work we both had ahead of us?

G: Well when you told me that you had a trainer in the past and you had lost so much weight I thought, Shit! I have to live up to that expectation or do better, so I was very keen. I love helping people so this was a great way for me to help you. I had everything planned out for at least a month and as I was training you, I saw how easily you were getting results. You never quit, but having said that, there were many times when you did want to quit.

S: Yep, there sure were.

G: I was happy that I took you on because it was a challenge for me and also a challenge for you too, Steve.

S: Although most of my success has been through Herbal products, intense fitness training has made a massive contribution to that success. How would you say that your training has helped in my success?

G: Steve, training is essential, you have to train. If you're not going to eat well then there is no point training. Yes, the Herbal products have had a massive impact obviously. They've helped you a lot, but it's also made you realise that training comes along well together with eating, nutrition and things like that. Training has made you a much fitter and stronger person.

S: Am I one of the biggest clients you have ever had?

G: Not anymore so well done! But yes, at the time you were my biggest client. I now have a client who is bigger than you, but you have been my biggest achievement and my number 1 client. In combination with the Herbal products and my training, you've lost over 30kgs, which is a massive deal for me.

S: Ok I have to ask you this George, what was your first impression of me before you were my trainer?

G: Well Steve, I have taken on a fair few clients. Some of them have been keen and others have just tried it and then given up. When I first saw you I was like "Is this guy serious"? I wanted you to be serious and see how you go, and you did, you put everything in it and so did I. My first reaction was *wow*, you put everything into that first session and that made me realise the type of person that you were and it made me keen to keep on training you in the long term.

S: I've lost over 30kgs. How do you feel knowing that your training has helped me achieve this success?

G: I feel awesome to have been a part of it all. It's great to see that my time and your time hasn't gone to waste and we have actually achieved something. 30kgs is a massive deal, it's just *wow*, I can't even explain it, I'm glad that I had that impact on you.

S: I started training with you back in November 2012, remind me again about my very first training session with you.

G: Well I didn't want to do too much to start with, but I also didn't want to do too little either. I wanted to make you do that extra bit to make you realise, shit, look where I'm at. I knew then that it was going to be tough and I wanted you to realise and understand that. I then, slowly, started introducing stuff that you didn't like doing so you could start getting better at them. Push ups, for example, you hated them, you couldn't do many push ups at the start, recently we've done about 75 push ups in 1 minute and that's a big deal. We've practised them and you complained a lot *(laughs)*.

S: Shut Up!

G: Well you did Steve. You kept saying, "I can't do it, you're not helping etc." but here we are now almost a year later and, well the results speak for themselves.

S: So I had my first progress measurements 6 weeks after I started training with you. You measured me on my first session and then 6 weeks later. After my first 6 weeks we can both honestly say that I delivered some pretty impressive results. How did you feel when you saw how happy and proud I was of the success?

G: *I was rapt, big time!* Seeing people happy makes me happy and especially knowing that I've helped them all because they trusted me. I mean, you trusted me to handle all this stuff, you lost 7cm off your waist in 6 weeks which, if you break it down, is like 1cm a week and that's a massive deal. You listened to everything I told you and it all paid off. You've done well mate.

S: Thanks! So what are some of the things that we cover in a typical 1 hour session of personal training?

G: Ok, well let's talk about a typical 'endurance' session. I time you so that we could do about 20 exercises for 1 minute each and 2–3 sets of those. I have to tell you though, they are intense, and you know that from doing them yourself, some of them you hate and others you love. You just push through it and that's all.

S: George, after three months of working with you, I was inspired by you and your whole attitude towards me and fitness. It was then that I too signed up to be a personal trainer at AIF. How did it make you feel knowing that you had that impact on me?

G: Steve, again I was rapt. To know that I had that impact on you made me proud; it makes me more proud because now you too want to help people just like I did. You're going to be in your own position now, helping other people who were in your shoes.

S: What have been some of my results with you since I started training? By that I mean, what's the heaviest weight I can lift, how many push-ups for instance?

G: Ok well first of all, your push-ups, at the start you hated them didn't you?

S: Yeah I did.

G: When you first walked in here, I made you do push-ups and you did them on your knees, you could barely do 8 of them. You would do 5 of them then pause, then another 5 and pause, but now, on your toes, you can get about 75 push-ups in 1 minute. With the bench press you have been lifting between 60–70kgs which is excellent. We also do what we call "the plank" and you can do that for 3 minutes and that's awesome. These exercises, when you first got here, you hated them all. To actually be able to do them now with such high reps is good.

S: How often do I attend personal training sessions with you and how long do the sessions usually go for?

G: You see me 3–4 times a week and we train for 1 hour. So that's 4 hours a week worth of training. I love it and I know you do too.

We usually train in the mornings; you get here early and then head off to work.

S: How would you describe my transformation over the last 12 months, from the first time that I walked into the gym until now?

G: Oh my God, I can't even begin to comprehend any of it.
When you first walked in here I thought *wow*, this is going to be a massive challenge. After your first 6 weeks when you lost 7cms off your waist I thought, *yes!* This is definitely going to work, your pushing yourself to achieve these results. You started eating healthy and I think Herbal products and your cousin helped you with that a lot. It's been an amazing transformation and I've enjoyed watching you disappear right before my eyes, it's insane. The most important things that have changed are your confidence, and your self-esteem, you're a completely different person now. Just watching you drop from 130kgs to now under 100 has been an amazing transformation that I just can't believe. Massive difference Steve, your personality is great and you're half the size you were when you first walked in here.

S: Looking back on everything that we have done, what can you say has been my biggest achievement in training specifically?

G: The most important thing I would say is your perseverance. You didn't always like the exercises that I was giving you, but you did love the results that you were getting from them. You kept persevering and kept going; you had the determination and because you loved the result that's why you have kept going. You also trusted me to train you and that's important to have that relationship with someone. You enjoy coming here and I enjoy training you. You've learnt to love it and that's the part I like the most, the fact that you love it, it's now part of your daily routine. You don't think of it as "Oh shit, I have to train now", you actually enjoy it.

S: What's been the toughest thing about training me?

G: It's been hard, but not tough. I think the hardest or the toughest thing about training you was making you do the exercises that you hated such as push-ups, which you're now great at I might add.

S: And what's been the easiest thing about training me?

G: The fact that you're always consistent. You always come to your sessions and you always make sure that you fit four of them in each week. There has never been a session where you couldn't be bothered showing up, the only exception has been if you were sick or in an emergency. That's been the easiest thing, knowing that you'll show up.

S: I already know the answer to this next question, but I'm never tired of hearing it. Are you proud of my success?

G: *Yes!* Very much, you're my number one client and I have enjoyed training you from Day 1. You've achieved the best results from me, I mean you have done all this on your own; I just trained you and told you what to do. Steve, I absolutely love training you, it's fun and I'm very proud.

S: Do you think that I will be a great role model and inspiration to other people who have been in my situation?

G: Yeah of course. You have the determination and you're always going to persevere to what you want. You said you were going to lose this much weight and you did it. You're on the right track and by the time you reach the end of your journey, hopefully in the next few months, we will get to where you want to be. You're definitely going to help people because you have an interest in dieting and exercise, so you can now show people that and help them along their journey. You're really determined and that's what I love about you.

S: I will be a qualified personal trainer soon and I'll go out there and pursue my own career, and obviously I'll never forget what we both have achieved together. Do you think that we can still keep in touch, keep a close friendship, exchange notes *(laughs)* and all that?

G: Yeah of course. That would be great; I don't see this as the end. I don't see it as you just coming here to train and then going home. It's not like that at all; we'll still keep in touch for sure. If you feel that you can train on your own then that's great, but I'll always be there to help and support you further. We've built a great relationship over the past year and it's been good.

S: Do you think I'll be a good personal trainer and why?

G: Absolutely, I think you'll make a great trainer because you've been trained by me *(laughs)*.

S: Oh get over yourself dude *(laughs)*.

G: You listen to what I say, hopefully that's rubbed off on you somehow. You have come so far, people are going to want to be trained by you because it's not just some random person off the street, you've worked hard for it and you'll be awesome.

S: I am nearing the end of my weight loss journey, and as I prepare for Part 2 and perhaps the next 6 months, what do you have in store for me in regards to training?

G: Steve, you've lost so much weight, the way I work and the way I help people get results is with a lot of resistance training.

We are going to be hitting the weights a lot harder and doing a lot more running. We are going to keep losing that weight until you get to your goal. It's going to be hard core and we're not going to stop, that's all I can say, so watch out, because those weights are going to be coming your way.

S: Finally, what would you like to say to me as we look forward to next few months when I finally reach my goal?

G: Steve, whatever you're doing, just keep doing it. It's been an awesome 12 months for me just as much as it has been for you. Just don't stop, just because you reach your goal, doesn't mean it all has to end there. Just set yourself new goals and keep trying to achieve them and then you'll complete your journey and feel awesome about yourself. So far in these 12 months you have done everything that I've asked and it's not over yet, we are going to keep going. Well done, I'm very happy and proud of you Steve.

S: Thank You.

Chapter 17

The First Training Session

By December 5th, 2012 I had lost a massive 20kgs on the Herbal products combined with my intense fitness training. The following photos are my progress shots. I had been taking the Herbal products for just over two months. These results are also after one month of intense fitness and personal training.

For the first time in almost 12 years the bulge in my stomach had started to fade away. My face had slimmed down and my upper arms where getting bigger due to all the weight training and just so slightly, my once skin tight singlet top, which at the time of this photo was a size 4XL or 120cm, was now loose and baggy.

Three days later, Saturday December 8th, 2012 I attended a family wedding with my Mum. By the weekend I had lost another kilo, taking my total loss to 21kgs, thanks to the combined efforts of the Herbal products and intense fitness training 4 times a week for 1 hour.

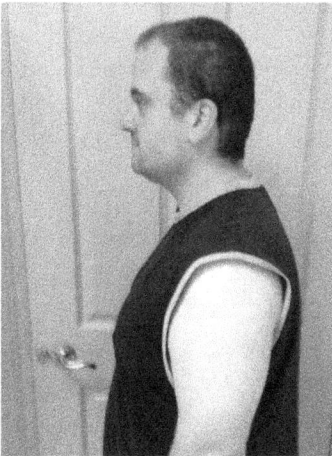

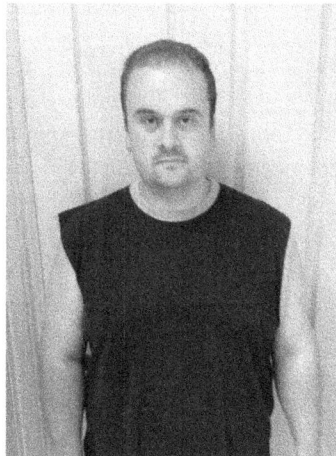

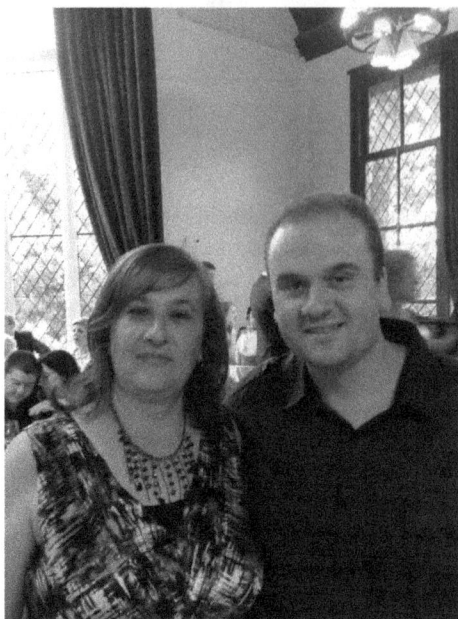

Mum and me at a family wedding on December 8th, 2012.
It was a great achievement losing 21kgs in 3 months.

December 21st, 2012. It was 4 days before Christmas and time for my first (six week) round of measurements from personal training. The following chart shows my progress after six weeks of personal training combined with the Herbal products and very strict dieting.

Week	Chest	Upper Arm	Calf	Waist	Hips	Thighs
1	124.5cm	40cm	49cm	131cm	121cm	68cm
6	120.5cm	39cm	48cm	124cm	117cm	71cm
Difference	- 4cm	- 1cm	- 1cm	- 7cm	- 4cm	+ 2cm

The massive difference here was the 7cm loss in my waist/stomach area, clearly showing that I was on the right track, eating right and exercising regularly. The 2cm gain in the thighs was due to weight training, which is normal in any form of exercise, especially when most sessions are cardio and you are using your legs. Two of my four sessions are cardio and the other two sessions focus on weights.

It was a great way to mark the end of 2012. I had lost 25kgs, my new body was finally starting to take shape and I was pleased with the results I had achieved so far. Even after massively pigging out on Christmas and New Year's Day, and having a couple of days off training with no exercise, I only managed to put on 1 kilo. Considering the amount of food I had eaten, 1kg was quite a pleasant surprise. During the month of January I continued training 3–4 times a week except for the week when George took his holidays.

Throughout January I maintained the weight loss and training consistently and continued to deliver some great results.

Chapter 18

Three Months Personal Training and Herbal Products

January came and went, February had arrived and summer had well and truly kicked in. I hated the heat and was dreading my training sessions in summer. Thankfully, my sessions were always in the morning at 8am so I generally missed the heatwave before it really kicked in.

February 1st, 2013 I had my next set of measurements; we were at the 12 week mark. After three months on the Herbal products and personal training I had achieved some more amazing results. The chart below shows the results I have delivered in total since I started the Herbal products and personal training.

Week	Chest	Upper Arm	Calf	Waist	Hips	Thighs
1	124.5cm	40cm	49cm	131cm	121cm	68cm
6	120.5cm	39cm	48cm	124cm	117cm	71cm
12	115cm	37cm	47cm	119.5cm	113.5cm	65cm
Difference	5.5cm	2cm	1cm	4.5cm	3.5cm	6cm
Total Diff.	- 9.5cm	- 3cm	- 2cm	- 12cm	8cm	- 3cm

I was amazed; 5 months into my weight loss journey I had achieved massive success. A loss of 32kgs and for the first time in over 12 years I was finally back in the double digits weighing 99kgs. After 5 months on my diet, 3 months on the Herbal products and personal training, the new me was finally taking shape and I was looking pretty good.

I never thought I would ever get rid of the big and baggy clothing, it was the best feeling, knowing that I no longer had to wear 'fat clothes'. It's amazing what I achieved with a lot of dedication and hard work. That's the difference in my stomach after five months. A great achievement that I am proud of and I have now finally got rid of those big pants.

On February 16th, 2013 I attended a seminar about the Herbal products at a convention centre in Bulleen with my cousins Chris and Suzi. We were joined by the man who started this journey for us all; former AFL Carlton footballer, Anthony Koutoufides, and many others who were a part of the Herbal products team.

The rest of February was tough, I had hit a major plateau, I wasn't losing any weight and I hadn't changed anything in my diet. I was still eating properly, still exercising and continued with the Herbal products. I was constantly texting Suzi, making sure that I was still doing everything correctly. She wanted to know what I was eating so I told her everything. George had been telling me certain foods that I should be eating in conjunction with my exercising, such as protein products, and salads. These would help with my training and help with the gain in muscle. Suzi had been doing this program for so long now and she had learnt what foods we should be eating and was able to write up a meal plan for me to help me get over the plateau.

The thing I actually found hard was getting into the habit of following the food plan. I had been doing so well on my own that I was too scared to change it in case I did something wrong. Suzi and I discussed the food plan and I took it home with me that night.

The food plan was documentation and a plan of the meals that I would be eating and at what times. For breakfast I usually had cereal, and a morning snack was a piece of fruit, like an apple. For lunch I usually had a meal replacement shake blended with fruit like strawberries. An afternoon snack was usually another piece of fruit or a protein bar and my dinner was usually a colourful meal. A colourful meal was a salad which consisted of lettuce (green), tomato (red), onion (white), capsicum (yellow) and olives (black).

The hardest part was eating late at night; I was always awake past midnight and always hungry before I went to bed. As a way to beat my hunger and stop having late night snacks before going to bed, I made myself a fruit smoothie. I used my meal replacement shakes and added ice and fruit to make it thicker so that I would be full.

Following this meal plan was essential to my fitness program, as it helped me keep fit and healthy. Exercising was one thing, but I also needed to eat healthy because I had so much weight to lose.

By following the food plan, I put an end to my plateau and lost 2 kilos the first week I was on it. After that, I managed to get back on track and started losing about a kilo a week following the food plan.

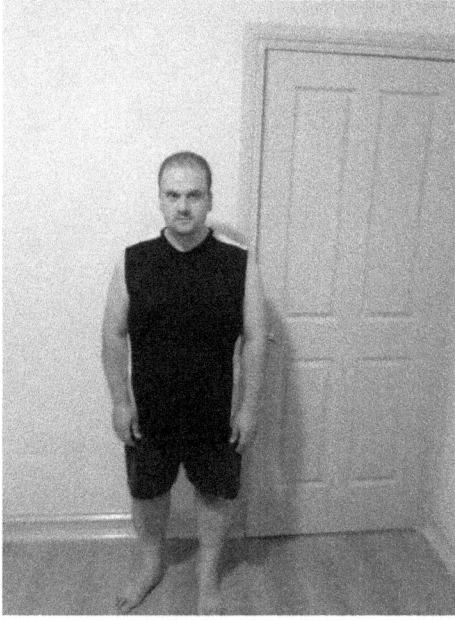

Chapter 19

Anthony Koutoufides

Throughout my life I've been fortunate enough to meet some very inspiring, dedicated and special people. Many of these people have been influential in my life, in one way or another.

As I was on the road to discovery, my cousins Chris and Sue formally introduced me to a very inspirational and dedicated man. The man, who introduced me and many others to these wonderful Herbal products that are today, used by millions around the world. A man who is my role model, my inspiration, my coach and former AFL Carlton footballer, Anthony Koutoufides.

I never really followed football and in my entire life I have only ever been to one live football match. Although I am a Collingwood supporter, I had obviously seen and heard about Anthony through the media and watching football games on the TV.

I first met Anthony in February 2013 at a seminar for the Herbal products which was held in Bulleen. I attended the seminar with my cousins Chris and Sue so that I could get a better insight into these products. I had only ever spoken to Anthony once previously and that was via Facebook and even then it was to discuss my progress on the products and the results that I was achieving.

I remember speaking to Anthony during a coffee break. Sue officially introduced us and we started talking. Since retiring from AFL Football, Anthony has kept himself busy holding weekly Fit Clubs and promoting the Herbal products. Anthony also plays the role of lifestyle coach to many others out there who are new to these Herbal products and have also started their own journey to weight loss.

I was fortunate enough to sit down and interview Anthony during my transformation through weight loss. We spoke about how he was introduced to these Herbal products and also spoke about what else he had been up to since leaving AFL football back in 2007.

Steve: Anthony, thanks for taking the time to speak to me.

Kouta: No problem.

S: So you started with Carlton Football Club back in 1990, what made you want to be a professional footballer?

K: Well as a young kid I had a dream, and it was to either be an athlete, Olympian or a footballer. At the age of 17 Carlton offered me a contract, so I decided at that stage to take up football full-time.

S: You retired from professional football in 2007. What have you been up to since then?

K: Well I've done a few things; I was a part of a TV show called *Gladiators*, I've been doing a bit of media work as well as appearing as a contestant on *Dancing with the Stars*. I've also worked for a car finance company, so I've done various things. Over the last few years however, I've found my passion again and I love to help people and I found out about these Herbal products. I got onto these products myself after being quite ill and seeing doctors. There was just no solution to what the doctors were telling me Steve, and that's when I started taking these Herbs that changed my life forever. Since I found the product I've worked extremely hard with the company and I have a belief that this product can help millions of people around the world.

S: Anthony, tell us a little more about your role at the Lifestyle Centre.

K: Steve, at the centre we basically help people. We are helping them health-wise and financially also. My role as a leader, is to help people in that way. It's my job to help people who are unhealthy and who want to get healthy. I can help them there and then financially if they want to earn some extra money, I can also help them with that.

S: I got started on the Herbal products through my cousins Chris and Sue, and they got onto them from you. But how did you find out about the product?

K: As I mentioned earlier Steve, a friend of mine had been involved with the company that distributes the product for a long time and he was a Carlton supporter and he told me about it. At first I was really sceptical about it, I think the way I was feeling I was like, you know what, I'll just give this a try. I did not think for one second that it was going to help change the way that I was feeling, and I think about five days into the program was when it did actually change the way I was feeling. Before taking the Herbs I was sleeping 11 hours a night and even sleeping throughout the day, Steve I literally couldn't even get out of bed. I was fatigued and tired and I had a lot of health issues, got onto this product and after five days it completely changed my life. So that's how I got on it.

S: How long have you been on the products, Anthony?

K: Just over 2 years now Steve, I started taking them back in February 2011 after being ill for about a year and I haven't missed a day. I swear by them and the more I take them, the better I feel.

S: Can you tell us what have been some of the results that you have achieved as a result of these products?

K: Well before the Herbs Steve, I was running 6.4kms in about 29–30 minutes; I was ill at that stage. That was on a good day, and then within three weeks of being on the program I got my time down to 26.5 minutes. Then I started to get a bit busy, I was travelling overseas and I was gone for about three weeks. When I returned, I had a little bit of training and I decided to give it another go. I ran the circuit in 25 minutes 40. To me, even when I was playing AFL footy, I don't think I ever ran that sort of time, but in saying that, I was specifically training to run 6.4kms. I know that personally, I've never run that sort of time before and I recovered from the training sessions very well.

Another thing, I have an arthritic shoulder that I have had problems with for the last 15 years and somehow, miraculously it has recovered and I don't feel the pain like I have in the past.

S: It's been a few months now and I've lost over 35kgs with the Herbal products combined with intense fitness training. What can you say about my success so far?

K: The thing that I admire about you Steve is that you took it upon yourself and you wanted to change your life. You wanted to change the way that you were feeling. Obviously you weren't feeling good before starting on the program, but by losing weight, you started to get confident, fitter and healthier. Steve, I think to be able to achieve that, it's all really about you. Yes, sure Sue and your personal trainer have been a massive part of your transformation and they have been there for support. Everyone needs support and that's what we do as health coaches; we support the person. However, at the end of the day it's up to the person, they need to be dedicated and sacrifice a lot of things to achieve their goals.

S: Now Anthony, you know that you have been one of my role models and also one of many people that have inspired me to take this journey to lose weight and have a healthier lifestyle. How does that make you feel?

K: Steve. Honestly I'm honoured, I really am. I don't feel like I've done anything out of the ordinary and I am really honoured to hear that. I don't see it that way, I see myself as doing everything right in life and I try to set the right example for people. Genetically, I may be better off than the majority of people, but I still take my health very seriously. When I saw my father ill (who passed away many years ago now), that was when I realised how important the value of health is to people. When he was ill, all he could do was think about himself and he forgot about his family. I mean you know what it's like Steve when you're not feeling well.

S: Yep.

K: It's important. There are a lot of health problems out there, but I believe we can help these people if they give us a chance. It's up to the individual.

S: The Herbal products are being used in over 88 countries around the world and by over 65 million people. What makes the product so successful?

K: Well, it's designed by the best doctors in the world and they spend something like over $100m a year on research and development. They have their own lab at the University of California in LA. They have a Nobel Prize winning doctor working for them as well as another doctor that got voted best doctor in America. The company has been going for over 33 years and they discovered Cellular Nutrition. These things get into the cells and change your life. They are the most wonderful product, backed by the best research and doctors in the world and manufactured by them. Seed to feed, we know everything that goes on with this product, so when I get it, I know I feel very comfortable to take a product instead of just buying it off the shelves. Not only that, you get personal coaching with your health coach as well so they can help you on your way. You're not just buying it off the shelf and taking it home and not knowing what to do with it, there are people there to coach you.

S: What can you recall about the first time you saw me face to face when you finally saw, for yourself, the results I had achieved?

K: When did I first meet you face to face, Steve?

S: It was at the Seminar in Bulleen.

K: Oh yeah! Right, well, obviously remarkable results, Steve. I could see the transformation from where you were to where you are now and *wow*, what can I say? I admire someone like you. You wanted to do something with your life in my opinion. I don't know why people wouldn't want to give this a go. I just don't understand it. I admire you for going, yep, I want to do this, and you know what, has the last 12 months been worth it for you? 100% it has. You can now look back and go yeah sure there were tough times, like anything in life, but you keep pushing through it and at the end is that pot of gold as we call it.

S: You briefly answered this but, although I haven't known you all my life, you have seen my transformation through Facebook, photos. How does it make you feel, knowing that other people as well as myself, are achieving results from these Herbal products?

K: Steve I feel thrilled. When I get a phone call from someone in WA who has Crohn's disease calling me and says "Kouta, thanks very much you've changed my life forever." Mate is there anything better in life? I've had a lot of supporters who have admired me playing footy, but now to hear this, I was over the moon to hear it. The doctors probably would have told him that there was nothing they could do about it and you're going to be in pain for the rest of your life.

However, we had the solution here that could help. I love it.

S: Were you reluctant to try the product at first?

K: 100%. If I was feeling good, I may not have tried it because I was a believer in food, but then I lost my belief in food when I got ill. I was training and eating organic food and I thought I was eating correctly and I still got sick, so of course I was reluctant, but the way I felt, I just wanted to give it a go when I heard all the background information on it, that's the only reason why I did.

S: How has it changed you Anthony?

K: You know what Steve, I love my life now. I have clarity in my mind, I sleep peacefully, I know I am getting all the right nutrients and at 40, I am recovering well and I feel young. I'm getting compliments all the time. How do you beat that? I don't know. But when people go *wow*, you are looking good, you look healthy. We are not just losing weight and looking unhealthy, we are losing weight and our skin looks younger. Internally your muscles are better, it's just an amazing product.

S: Being an athlete you were always fit and active. How important is exercise and a healthy lifestyle to you?

K: It's a part of my life Steve. It's always been a part of my life. The year that I was sick I was extremely down on myself. I don't know if I can call it depression, I try not to use that word, but it's not nice when someone has been so active and has gone through that. Sport to me, and being healthy, has been a part of my life as a young kid. I have always been outdoors and I guess to a lot of people I was known as *'The Body'* when I played AFL. I don't want people to see me overweight and putting on weight. I want them to look at me and go *wow*, your still looking good.

S: This goes without saying, but I've achieved massive success in such a short period of time and I have you and the Herbal products to thank for that. The important question here is what advice can you give to people like me, who are overweight, embarrassed with their image and have tried all sorts of diets with no success?

K: If they haven't tried this product, I would say try it. It's proven worldwide, it is the biggest healthy nutritional product in the world and just give it a go. I don't know how many people come to me, and people who have struggled to lose weight on other diets, and they get on here and all of a sudden the results are so evident. All I can say is; give it a go for sure.

S: Are you proud of the success that these Herbal products have brought you and the people that you have surrounded it with?

K: Yes! 100%. This company is all about caring for people and I think that is very important in life for personal development. If they are achieving things, then we are achieving things too, so that's a great feeling for us. We are backed by supportive people and they are seeing people get healthier. Some people want to get wealthy too and this company provides both.

S: Finally Anthony, you inspired me to take this incredible journey. Are you proud of me and the success with the Herbal products?

K: Of course I am proud of you. I'm proud of you and the person that got you on the product (Sue). I'm proud of everyone that has been involved, by me inspiring others to achieve their goals it makes me a happy person. I still have a lot more to achieve, I am going to go out there and promote this product more and get people fit and healthy. As years go by there are going to be more unhealthy people out there. We have an obesity epidemic in Australia and we feel like there is so much for us to achieve out there; we are going to do the very best that we can to do that.

S: Thanks Anthony.

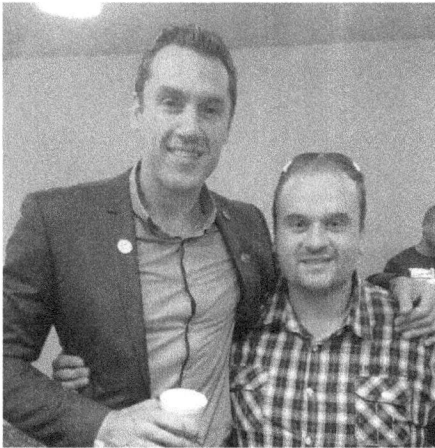

Anthony Koutoufides and me in February 2013.

Chapter 20

AIF

The Australian Institute of Fitness

George had made a massive impact on my weight loss and because of his intense fitness training, I was achieving my results. The next decision I made was perhaps the best decision I had ever made in my life. I realised that as a result of my success, it was now time for me to start sharing that with other people and to start helping others achieve the same success that I did.

On February 13th, 2012 I drove down to Williamstown where I enrolled into a full-time course at AIF, (Australian Institute of Fitness), as a personal trainer. That was something I thought I would never hear myself say, ever. But I did! It was actually happening and my first class started on April 10th, 2013, the day of my 32nd birthday.

The Australian Institute of Fitness is better known as the institute where celebrity personal trainer, Michelle Bridges of *Biggest Loser* fame, did her training as a Master Trainer.

I got my enrolment pack and left the building feeling excited and nervous at the same time. I was about to start a new journey, a journey to help others and that was the best feeling, knowing that I was now on my way to a happier and healthier lifestyle while helping others.

On my birthday, at 4pm I started my induction for the course at the Bundoora campus. I met my fellow class mates or 'friends' as they are called and we learnt more about the Institute and what was going to be expected of the course over the next six months. I was thrilled, walking out of that building knowing that in a few months I was going to be fully qualified. I was finally going to help other people with their struggles, just like George was able to help me with mine.

My first official day of classes was Wednesday 24th April and I attended classes two days a week on Wednesdays and Thursdays from 9am to 4pm. After not being at school for over 15 years, it was difficult to grasp the concept of trying to learn how to study again. I can honestly tell you all, I loved the course and learnt many things that I never knew before and look forward to helping many others out there when I am qualified.

I had been working in retail almost half my life. I never imagined ever leaving, as it was the only thing I knew how to do. I never imagined that I would find myself helping others to get fit and lose weight. After taking this incredible journey, I realised that it wasn't a matter of wanting to help other people, but rather needing to help them. It was time for a change and my change was a career as a personal trainer.

On Friday 8th, March 2013 it was time for some more measurements. The table below shows my results after approximately 18 weeks; four and a half months of personal training and five months on the Herbal products.

Week	Chest	Upper Arm	Calf	Waist	Hips	Thighs
1	124.5cm	40cm	49cm	131cm	121cm	68cm
6	120.5cm	39cm	48cm	124cm	117cm	71cm
12	115cm	37cm	47cm	119.5cm	113.5cm	65cm
18	116.5cm	38cm	48cm	116.5cm	113cm	67cm
Difference	1.5cm	1cm	1cm	3cm	.5cm	2cm
Total Diff.	- 8cm	- 2cm	- 1cm	- 14.5cm	-8cm	- 1cm

My biggest loss was once again around my waist, 14.5cm down in just under 5 months. Although the other areas all gained, this was perfectly normal. I was gaining muscle because of all the weight training and as a result of this my upper arms and chest were expanding.

Everything was on track and I continued to lose weight at a steady rate. There's no denying that by this stage, I was rapt with what I had achieved. Everything was falling into place and I was doing really well.

Sue and George were both extremely proud of my success. I was looking and feeling a lot healthier and I was a much happier person. I delivered some pretty impressive results from my Herbal check-up as well.

Body Fat Range	% Body Water Range	Muscle Mass	Physique Rating	BMR	Basic Metabolic Age	Bone Mass	Visceral Fat
39	47.4	69.4	3	3501	46	3.6	22
37.2	48.1	68	3	3406	46	3.5	20
37.2	48.2	65.9	3	3295	46	3.4	19
36.1	48.7	64.9	3	3234	46	3.4	18
34.7	49.2	66.4	3	3298	46	3.5	17

After five months, compared to when I first started on the Herbal products, there was a massive difference that personal training, healthy eating and exercise has made to achieving my success.

My Visceral Fat was **22**, it's now **17** = **ALARMING**
My Metabolic Age = **46**, this will take time to change.
My Physique Rating = **3** which is **Solidly-built**

Age	Excellent	Healthy	Medium	Obese
20–24	10.8	14.9	19.0	**>23.3**
25–29	12.8	16.5	20.3	**>24.3**
30–34	14.5	18.0	21.5	**25.2**

Compared to my results at the start of my weight loss journey, the key areas of success have been the Body Fat Range and the Visceral Fat; the two dominant areas which would have caused severe health issues. If we break it down it reads the following:

My age is **32** and I started with a Body Fat Range of **39**. It has now come down to **34.7**. The Visceral Fat, when I started, was **22**. It has now dropped to **17** which still = **OBESE**, but I am almost out of the ALARMING range which is over 13.

Hard work, determination, dedication and support sum up the main factors to my success. I was surrounded by many negative elements in my personal life which had a huge impact on my weight loss journey previously. I needed to eliminate myself from that equation if I had any hope of success, and I did.

As I near the end of this amazing journey in weight loss, I have come to learn that not everyone is supportive. It plays a major part and without it, I would have failed. I almost did. Not having that support made my journey tough, but it also made me more determined to go on and succeed.

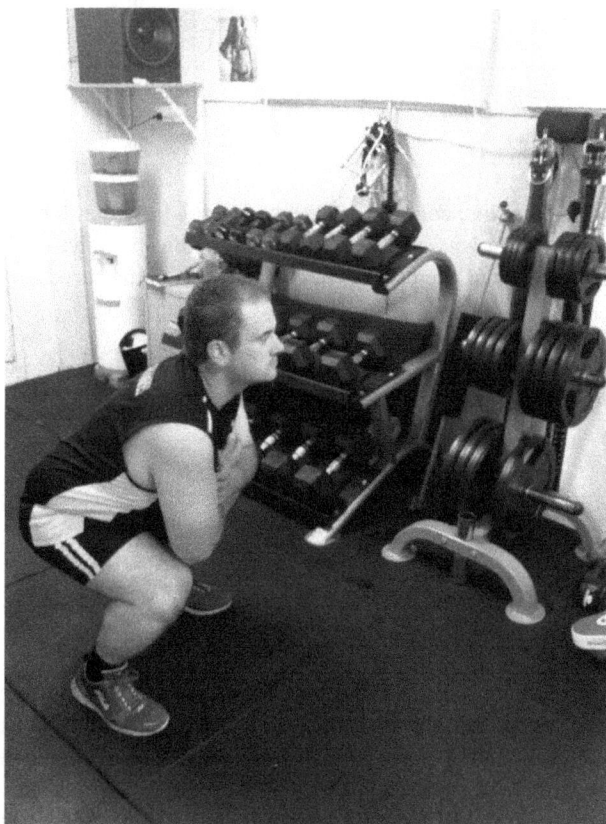

Squats are a great leg exercise that really works your quads. The most important thing to remember is to have your back straight at all times. Not only is this the correct technique, it also prevents any back or spinal injuries. Generally aim for a consistency of about 30 seconds to 1 minute for optimal results.

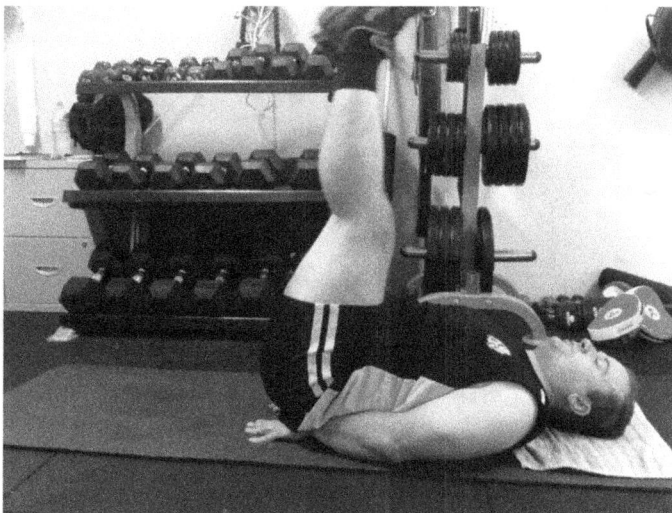

Leg raises. This is great for any abs workout. Once again, make sure you are on a flat surface and your back is straight and your legs are stretched out all the way. Have your hands out to your side rather than under your bum. It's harder, much harder in fact, but you are getting a more thorough workout. Try and aim for a consistency of about 30 seconds to 1 minute for great results.

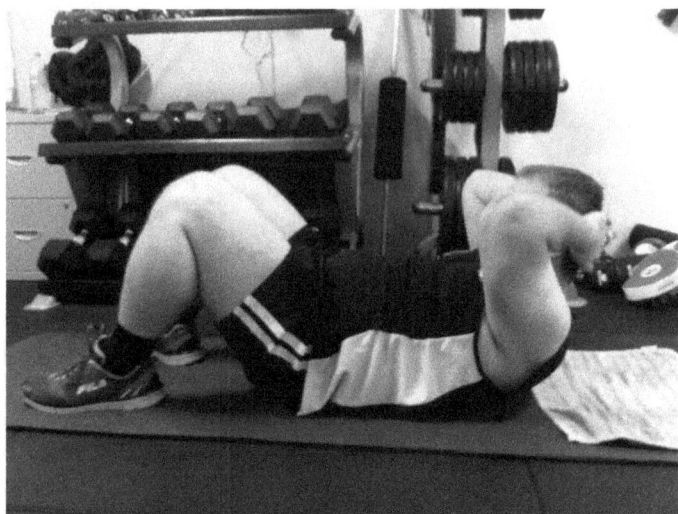

Sit ups. This is one of the best forms of exercise for your abs. With everything else, make sure back is straight and you are on a flat surface. Place your hands behind your head and hold them together. Bring your knees up and then bring your elbows to your knees. Remember to breathe out on the way up.

Chapter 21

My final interview is with a woman who has inspired me in many ways. She has taught me to fight, never give up and most importantly, not to give a shit about what anyone else might think. The one thing I always had a problem with, other than my confidence and self-esteem, was listening to what others thought about me.

Tina Gephart is an inspirational, dedicated and hardworking Mum who has always been there to support me no matter what the issue. I remember never having laughed so much in my whole life before meeting Tina. During the short time that Tina and I have worked together, we have become very close friends and remain in each other's lives.

Tina is not just a loyal and dear friend to me, but also my inspiration. She has watched me develop as a person over the last two and a half years and she has also been there for my entire transformation through weight loss. In early 2013 Tina decided, out of the blue, that she wanted to write her first novel. Not being an author, or having any experience in the field, Tina set out on her quest to write a best-selling novel. After three months of hard work and dedication, it was mission accomplished. Tina put all her ideas on paper and came up with not only a plot, but an ingenious story that I believe will one day be her very own best seller.

The beauty about Tina is that when she sets her mind to something, she does it. That was the kind of inspiration that I needed in my life to make sure that I succeeded. Tina also sees things like they are and I was no exception. Tina could always tell whenever there was something wrong with me. Even when I insisted there was nothing wrong, Tina wouldn't take no for an answer; she knew me better than that.

Having Tina around through a troubled time in my life, pushed me to fight through with a grim determination. She could always make me laugh, no matter how hard things got or how upset I was. She always made me feel better and was able to focus on the bright side of things.

Once again, friendship and loyalty between friends comes into play with this story. Tina's inspiration to write her novel was my inspiration to help me lose weight and start telling the world about my story, my troubles, and most of all, to start helping people who may be in similar situations.

Like Sue, Tina was always around after hours. Whenever I had a problem that I couldn't deal with on my own, I could always pick up the phone and give her a call or send her a text. Tina was available day or night to help me whatever way she could, even though she had no obligation.

As Tina got to know me a lot better, she too discovered that my weight and image were major contributing factors to my lack of self-esteem, confidence and negativity. As a result, she could see what it was doing to me. Tina could be having the crappiest day and still, she would find a way to make a joke about it all and act like nothing had happened. Having that sort of attitude around me took me out of my comfort zone.

I saw all the hard work and dedication that Tina was putting into her novel and this made me push myself harder to reach my goal as well. Working with Tina was the happiest time whilst I was at Village, and as I took this journey through weight loss and to complete my story, Tina watched me change into a different person.

As I started losing the weight everything was changing, and I am not just talking about the obvious changes. I was happier, I was a better person to be around and people started to actually appreciate me because of the path I had decided to take.

I have always seen Tina as an inspirational role model, mother, best friend, and (ouch), she slaps me for calling her my mother and making her sound old, so I guess sister will do. The woman I will always be proud to say that I know. Tina is the woman who inspired me to take this life changing experience and finally make a long-awaited transformation.

As I bid a teary farewell to Village Cinemas Doncaster and start my new venture at the Village Drive-Ins in Coburg, I had the opportunity to speak candidly with Tina as she talks to me in her first ever interview.

Tina talks to me about her life, her friends, her inspirations and writing her first novel. She also talks about how she has watched me develop over the past two and a half years into the person that I have become today, and about what the future may hold for her.

Steve: Tina first of all congratulations on the success of your first novel *A Twist of Fate*. The first question I want to ask you is what inspired you to write a book?

Tina: Well basically my friends and I were reading those trashy adult porn novels and that sort of genre, and in my mind, the females in those books were not represented in a way that I could relate to them. They were weak and fragile with negative personalities, clearly not somebody I could relate to. You know what Steve, it kind of started as a dare, I was saying to everyone that I could do this, I can write a book, sure, no worries. Then I put it out there and...*(pause)*, well once it's on Facebook you have to pull through *(laughs)*.

S: You have to go ahead and deliver once it's out there on Facebook.

T: Pretty much, once I say something, I follow through. I never had any aspirations to be an author, but that was what inspired me to write the book.

S: Ok so how did you and I first meet Tina?

T: I believe it was my second shift at Village in Gold Class. I started on as a Christmas casual. So it was either my second or third shift. That was back in November 2010.

S: What were your first impressions of me Tina?

T: Can I lie about that one?

S: No!

T: Ok. Um, it's hard to say Steve, at the time I was meeting a lot of people. When I first met you though, you were one of the first people that I definitely remembered. There were a few people whose names I wouldn't even remember. I think you were a little bit different than the others that were working there because you were a lot older and more mature. I definitely remembered you first off the rack. As far as my first impression...

S: **Now be nice** *(laughs)*.

T: Always. My first impression, I would say that you were definitely a hard worker, and very determined, very dedicated. So that would probably be my first impression of you Steve.

S: **You wrote your book in just over three months. How did you come up with the idea for such a great story?**

T: I guess for me, with anything, I kind of get something in my head and then I build on it. So I have always been blessed in a way that I can spin. I can elaborate upon, stretch and embellish. So I just had a basic idea about what I wanted the story to be about. Obviously they had to be strong, independent, focused women to a point, and obviously I was writing it to go up against all the other adult novels out there, so it was always going to have an exotic slant to it. I wanted it to be character based and driven so that you actually fall in love with the people in the story and not just the story itself. Having so many interesting characters in my life, I was able to draw from that inspiration and I just kind of built the story around that.

S: **Now, I have always called you my sister and you know that I speak very highly of you and your achievements. Are you proud of what you have achieved so far?**

T: Yes. Now Steve, let's be perfectly honest, you only call me your sister because you called me Mum once and I almost slapped you *(laughs)* so I guess sister will do. I think, Steve, I am my own worst critic. I am definitely proud of the book and proud of what I have achieved thus far, but I don't think it's all that I have left to give. I think that I definitely have more to achieve. I guess you can say that this makes me hungry for more success.

S: **I have always struggled with my weight and image as well as my personal life for many years, even long before you and I met. What can you say about my journey over the last few months?**

T: Well, ever since I have known you Steve, your weight has always been an issue for you. You were always on some kind of diet or trying something different, constantly yo-yoing, losing it, putting it on and all that. I think you became overly focused on the weight, rather than the issue which was an esteem issue for you I think. When I looked at you Steve, I didn't necessarily look at you as a fat person; I looked at you as someone who wasn't happy with himself. Since losing the weight, it's probably the most driven I have ever seen you. You set out to do something and you did it, you were consistent. Steve, that is something to definitely be proud of and a lot of people say that they are going to do stuff and they never do, so I take my hat off to you on that one.

S: Thank You. You have watched me develop over the years, even though it's only been a short time. Do you think my weight loss achievement has made me a different person and given me a better outlook on life?

T: Absolutely, like I said, before it wasn't just a weight issue, it was an esteem issue. It was a symptom of something else and I think since losing the weight you have actually proven to yourself that you can do something if you set out on a goal and follow through with it. I think that in turn, not only have you lost a shit load of weight, but I think it's had a positive impact on you. You have proven to yourself and everyone else, but mainly yourself, that you can do this and that will fold out onto anything else that you put your mind to. I think you now have a much healthier outlook on life, mentally I mean and not with food. I think you'll be great.

S: Weight loss has changed my life. Has writing a book changed your life?

T: Yes, definitely. Before writing the book I was working, I was a Mum; I was seeing my friends...

S: You are still primarily a Mum, though?

T: Yes, of course. I am still a Mum, and I still do see my friends and I am still working, but as I was growing up I never decided what I wanted to be. My resume reads like I am some sort of freak, because I didn't have a desire to do anything. Since writing the book and actually seeing it through to the end and having people read it, gives me pleasure and makes me feel proud. It has given me a direction and it is something that I can now see myself doing. If I could earn money from it I would definitely give up work in a flash. It is good for me in the sense that it has given me a focus and an outlet and that final "this is what I want to do".

S: During the time that you have known me, what would you say has been my biggest weakness?

T: Yourself. It always has been Steve. I would also say that you can self-sabotage and you do not believe in yourself. There have been many times when you and I have spoken and I would say to you that you need to look inside yourself. There is no one out there who thinks any of this of you, but yourself. I don't know if there is something deeper than that where people have been telling you that you were never worthy of anything and you chose to believe that yourself, but definitely your biggest weakness is you.

S: Ok, on the flip side, what would you say are my strengths?

T: Steve, you are loyal. Incredibly loyal, I do not, for a second, ever believe that you would do anything to any of your friends in a negative way. I believe that once you are friends, you are friends. That is rare these days. I think that people can be quite fickle with their relationships. You are also hard working, so that's also a good thing.

S: Looking back, through the time that you have known me, what can you say about this whole transformation in general?

T: Well the most obvious thing that comes to mind is of course the physical transformation. Watching you shrink before our eyes, honestly, I want the best for you Steve, I want you to succeed, as it gave me a lot of pleasure to see you doing this. I think other than the physical side of it, which is more visible to the eye, your outlook changed. You are a lot happier, things like buying a pair of jeans, I am sure was something that you couldn't do before. It's just been nice to see all these changes in you and taking ownership in what you have done and putting it out there. You post your pictures on Facebook and you share your transformation, that's something to be proud of. The old Steve would never have done that and just thought "oh well, who cares."

S: Back to you, you are currently working on the third and final novel in the series. How is that all going?

T: Of course it's back to me, what did you think this was, all about you? *(laughs)* The third book is *fantastic*, it's almost done. Initially it was hard and only because I was putting pressure on myself. With the first book no one really expected anything, I didn't expect anything of myself, I was just telling a story and that's all I wanted to do. I tried to make it funny, interesting and something that I would want to read. With book two, I put pressure on myself, because the first one was so good, I thought what happens if this one blows, what if people hate it. I wrote the first chapter, took a really long break and then I wrote the second chapter and again took another break, and then I finally thought to myself, this is stupid. If I don't want to do this I can put it away and not look at it, or I can do what I set out to do the first time, and that is to tell a good story and hope that people will read it and enjoy it. Since I have done that, since I took the pressure off myself, it has been amazing. It's been easier to write the characters this time around, I get to explore them a lot more, I'd be sitting there writing dialogue and I would just crack myself up because I hear their voices inside my head *(laughing)*. And not because I have multiple personalities Steve, let's make that perfectly clear for everyone out there ok?

S: Oh no of course not *(laughs)*.

T: It was much easier this time around. I am really enjoying it and I cannot wait. I really can't.

S: You and me both.

T: It's coming.

S: Tina, what do you think has helped contribute to your success?

T: The fact that I said I was going to do something and I did it. Whereas some people get distracted and they don't finish it. Some people don't put a lot of faith in me and think to themselves "Oh who does she think she is"? My theory is like, well you know what, I'm going to do it anyway. Having the right attitude, if you set your mind to it you can do it. Also the support of my beautiful friends and family, they have all been there cheering me on, that's also helped a lot. Knowing that people are behind me too, that gives me strength to keep pushing through.

S: Here's one for you, Tina, describe me in 10 words.

T: Seriously? Ok, well hard working, loyal, thoughtful, generous, extremely generous, happy, but only recently. In the past I would say you were clouded, funny...Um, that's all I've got sorry.

S: You had a dream and you pursued it. This also helped me achieve my success. How does it make you feel knowing that you inspired someone else to pursue their dreams?

T: Flattered. I feel flattered to think that what I have done has impacted someone else's life. I certainly didn't set out to inspire anyone, I know that's not very noble, but I didn't, I really didn't give that much thought to it. If I have had that effect on someone then that makes me feel amazing, that I had in some way helped them. I am just trying to be a good friend to you Steve and to make you the best that you can be. If you see me, leading by example and that in turn inspires you, whether it's me writing a book or at work, then that makes me feel good to know that I'm looking after you.

S: *(Laughs)*.

T: Not that you need looking after, but you know what I mean.

S: What advice would you give to people who have a dream?

T: First of all, do not listen to the haters. No matter what your dream is, there are going to be people who have negative thoughts and negative ideas and that's their problem not yours. You need to remove that negativity from your life and concentrate. Steve, there is no shame in failure, if you strive for something and you do not get there, at least you tried. If you sit around and criticize other people and you never try, then to me, that's the real disaster. At the end of the day no one is going to look at you and go, "oh that person tried to do something and they failed". They are going to forget the failures; they are only going to remember what you actually accomplished. If you have a dream, grab it with two hands and go for it, don't let anyone stand in your way.

S: Are you proud of my success as well as your own?

T: Yes! Of course, I am very proud of your success Steve. I am very proud that you have taken ownership and you are moving forward with positive changes in your life. If I, in any way, contributed to that then it makes me feel very proud. Even though sometimes I know that you can be afraid, you took that risk and that's amazing. As for my success so far, I have so much more to give and so much further to go. I don't sit around and go *wow*, this is fantastic, I see it as a small step. My goal now, is to get this book of mine published and to get it read by others. The money isn't that big a deal for me, but it would be nice *(laughs)*, let's be honest.

S: Yes, let's be honest.

T: I am just proud to be doing what I am doing and continue to be doing what I am doing, and hope that I am a good role model for my children and for people around me.

S: Do you think that I will be a good role model for others who are trying to lose weight and get healthy?

T: Absolutely. I think people will look at your voyage and see where you have come from and the journey that you have been on and I think it's important not to discount the failures prior. The fact that you have tried to lose weight in the past and haven't succeeded, or if you have succeeded, you put it back on, yet refused to give up. It's important for people to realise that. I think the other important factor is that you have had health issues and it hasn't been an easy ride for you. You have had other things that have impacted on your journey. It's easy for you to just say, yep I have had health issues and it's too hard I am not going to do it. I think now you can say: "Hey I've been where you have been, I've had this, or I've done that and I still managed to do it". I think that will give people a positive message and they will be saying: "Hey if he can do it, I can".

S: Finally, Tina what would you like to say to me as I approach the end of this chapter and say goodbye to Doncaster?

T: Definitely just continue to keep striving, although it's easy to get distracted. Sure people acknowledge what you have done and they praise you for it. But after a while, people stop saying it, and that makes you forget the awesome thing that you have achieved.

S: Which has happened.

T: Exactly, so don't lose sight of how far you have come, don't ever lose sight of that. Don't diminish what you have done either. Find something else to be hungry for Steve (and I don't mean food), I mean attitude. Find something else. Your first goal was to lose weight. Find something that you could not have done if you hadn't lost all this weight, whether it is a sport, or climbing a mountain, sky diving, or something completely different. Use your time and energy to achieve that goal, so you're constantly revisiting and revising, and then no matter what is going on in your life, you have to focus. That is what I would say to you, Steve; have a focus, lock it in, and just go forward, don't look back, in not looking back, remembering what's come before this time.

S: Thanks Tina.

Chapter 22

Setting the Record Straight

It's hard when there is something blocked up deep inside that just wants to come out but can't. Keeping things to myself, all these years, especially my sexuality has been difficult. It took me many years, well into adulthood, to realise that I definitely wasn't gay and wanted to be with a woman.

Coming out wouldn't be the right phrase to use as I am not gay, but having expressed how I felt at the time, was a way of coming out itself. Perhaps, I will always have that fear of being judged, even now, but setting the record straight and knowing which path I want to take is a huge load off my chest. Friends and family continue to support me the best way that they all can and that is by being there for me when I need them.

Finding true love and happiness is going to be the next challenging part of my journey. After facing many of my demons, this is yet another one that I have to face. A simple challenge, but yet so hard when I consider the way my life has been up until now.

My road to discovery and opening up about who I really am has been a painstaking journey I have had to endure. At 32 I could not ask for any more than what I have. I have my life, my health and the support of all my family and friends around me. Winning the lottery might help, but money isn't everything in life, by no means.

I never thought that I would ever start my own business and finally do something that I truly enjoy. Having worked in retail almost half my life, I always thought that I would stay there. But now, having that feeling of knowing that I will actually be helping people battle their toughest demons gives me great pleasure.

Being bullied as a child, and having to hide that inside for many years, has been a daunting experience. It's not easy to talk about and I know that many of my 'bullies' have moved on to become better, intelligent people living great lives. I also know that there are many out there who continue to live in that world of pity because it makes them feel good to see others hurting.

One thing that my life experiences have taught me is that life comes at us with many hurdles, hardships and challenges. Even now, at 32, I am still faced with many challenges in my life, some of which I may unfortunately, never get around to completing.

Health and fitness have become a major factor in my life. Knowing now that my fitness has improved substantially from where it was twelve months ago, gives me a healthier outlook on my life, not to mention a change of habits.

Sitting down every night for the past eighteen years or so and typing my thoughts on a blank computer screen has been an emotional journey. Coming home every night and expressing how you feel to a computer isn't easy, especially when it doesn't talk back to you.

As I close the chapter on this part of my life, I look back on the struggles and achievements of the last twenty years or so. I look back and reflect on what has been my journey and discovered that I could indeed take my life...One Step Further.

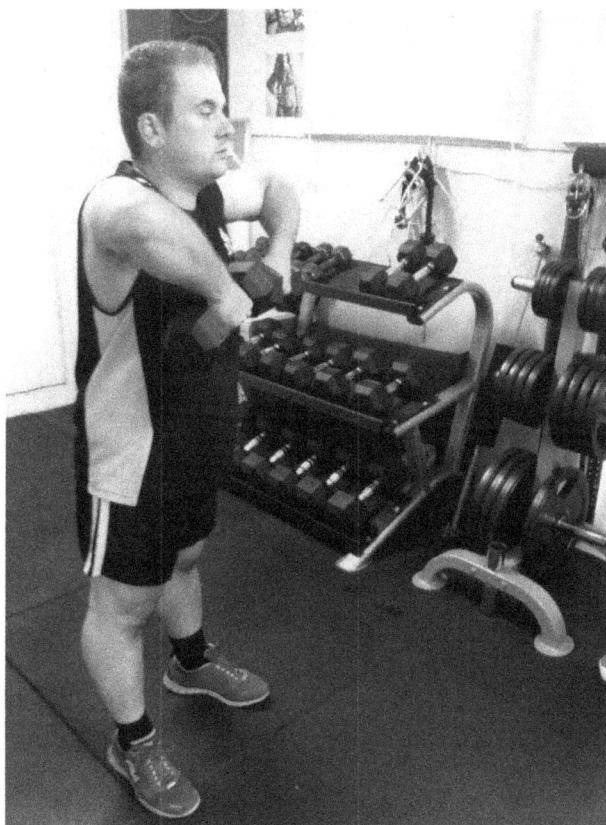

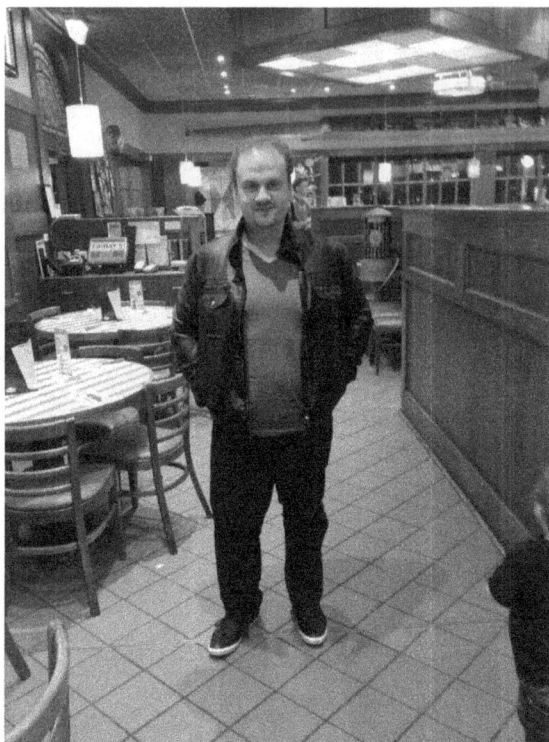

Acknowledgements

There are so many people who have really contributed to my life. All their support, comments, encouragement, compliments and believing in me from the start, have all got me to this point in my journey so far. I don't know how I could have achieved all this if it wasn't for these amazing people.

Firstly, to Paul Stanley for purchasing the very first copy of the book. Also to Liz Mirenzi, Amber Lane, Tina Alabakov, Daniela Crisafulli, Kristy Trafford, Marie, Tina Gephart, Nicole Foenander and Gino Giacobbe; a huge thank you to all of you for pre-purchasing your copies and supporting me on my journey to publish my first book.

Mum, Dad, Paul and Christopher, thank you for supporting me all my life and accepting the decisions I have made; the right and the wrong. This journey has been a challenging and life-changing experience and it has taught me about what is most important in my life; self-discovery. Thank you for all that you have done, I love you all deeply.

Catarina Fernandes is the one that got me started on this remarkable journey. Although our time working together was short and brief, she constantly kept a close watch on me and was always on my back every single day, keeping a close watch on everything I was eating. Thank you for getting me started on this incredible journey I will always be grateful to you.

My two incredible cousins (V) and (M) thank you both for your endless support throughout this entire experience. All your proof readings, edits, putting up with my constant texts and your feedback to help me get this novel published and out into the world. I love you both very much and words alone are not enough to express how much I appreciate all you have done for me. Thank you.

My extended family, over the years you have all seen me struggle with my weight, image and personal struggles and know how hard it has been for me. You have all supported me; this wouldn't have been possible without all your love and support.

To my dearest friends, Chris and Theresa Lindsay and their children Jayden and Cruze. They have all been there with me for this remarkable journey since the start, and continue to be there. I love you all very much and I cannot ask for better people in my life to share this experience.

Loretta Randhawa, you have been a part of my life for over 16 years, you are an amazing woman. You are my strength, rock, happiness and soul mate and I love you to bits. Thank you for always being you, the one that I will always love and treasure.

Jason and Rebecca Guthrie, who have stayed loyal to me for many years and remain my dearest friends, I thank you both for your constant support and kind wishes, I hope that one day I may be able to repay you.

Helen Harrop and Kylie Byrne, all your kind words of encouragement and your belief in me from the start is what has kept me going on for this long. You two will always be a part of me and this journey. You girls are my rocks as your endless love and support have pushed me all the way to my success and lifted my self-esteem and confidence.

My hot, inspirational 'sister' as I like to call her, Tina Gephart, for inspiring me to take this journey because she went and took one herself. Tina, you are an incredible woman who supports me in everything that I choose to do. I hope that you achieve the same success that I have and I wish you every happiness and great fortune.

Rebecca Andrews, for being there for me and putting me back in my place whenever I lose my way and for always knowing the right words to say.

Hayley Griffiths, the girl who always made my day. Hayley, your incredible love, support and constant words of encouragement have pushed me this far without wanting to give up. Thank you for being there for me and constantly striving for me to succeed.

Tom Brophy, what can I say? You are in every way shape and form the most incredible guy I know. You were there for me at a time when I was down and you continue to be the most amazing friend I could ever ask for.

My two special girls, Kim Dellevergin and Julie Sinclair, you girls always make me laugh and make me feel good about myself. I am very fortunate to have you both in my life to help me experience this incredible achievement. It's all your kind words, motivation and support that has got me this far and I love you both.

Anthony Koutoufides. You introduced my cousins Suzi and Chris Karakaltsas to the amazing Herbal products. If it wasn't for you telling her about this product I never would have found out about this amazing program, which has helped me and many others achieve amazing weight loss results so far.

Suzi, my attitude, new image, energy, love and dedication towards my new lifestyle has been due to all your support and consultations. I apologise for all the late night 'catch up's', the endless text messages and sometimes pointless, annoying phone calls at all hours of the night. No words will ever be enough to thank you for these remarkable results.

Nick Symeou, our time working together was brief, but if I had never met you, then I would not have been able to achieve much at all. Thank you for introducing me to the most amazing, motivated, inspirational, dedicated and hard working person I have ever met, your brother, my personal trainer and dear friend, George Symeou.

George, Wow! Mate, nothing can ever describe what I am feeling right now, and there is nothing that I could possibly say that you haven't heard me say to you already. Your hard work, attitude, personal experiences and intense training have brought me to this. You are an amazing person and a major motivation, I owe you so much. What you have turned me into over the last few months and the amount of time that we have put in together has made me accomplish this and given me the strength to carry on. All the endless hours of training and constant text messaging at all hours, to make sure that I am eating the right foods and exercising properly, has finally paid off. Thank you so much for being the most inspirational, supportive and patient man I have known and for turning me into who I am today. We achieved this together and we will continue to do so as this extraordinary journey is far from over.

Aly Walsh, for believing in me and never letting me give up whenever things got down. For helping me find my inner-self, supporting me, listening to me, putting up with my immense amount of text messages and emails at all hours and for being the incredible, hard working woman that you are. Thank you for publishing my first book.

Phil Dimitriadis, thank you for all your endless hours of editing and re-structuring this story to make it what it is now. Thank you for your time, loyalty, and amazing work, this would not have been possible without you.

Finally, to you, for reading my story. I hope that in some way this book will provide you with the confidence, hope and inspiration that you need to fulfil your dreams and speak out. Don't hold anything back and just go for it. Thank you for following my journey and supporting me by purchasing a copy of this book. Without all of this I could not have shared this journey with the rest of the world.

References

Goodrem, Delta. 'Born to Try', from the album *Innocent Eyes*, Sony Records, March, 2003

www.ingramcontent.com/pod-product-compliance
Lightning Source LLC
Chambersburg PA
CBHW072137020426
42334CB00018B/1846